I F'N HATE DEMENTIA

by
Ashley Ivy, MCD, SLP-CCC

Published by
SuburbanBuzz.com LLC
Texas, USA

First Edition: 2026

Printed in the United States of America

ISBN: 978-1-969877-03-2

DEDICATION

For the ones who show up
even when it hurts,
even when it's impossible,
even when it feels like the world has forgotten you.

For every caregiver —
family, friend, neighbor, spouse, child —
who loves someone through a disease
that does not love them back.

For the ones who sat beside hospital beds
and kitchen tables,
in silence and in chaos,
doing the work no one applauds.

For the ones who stayed
when it would have been easier to leave.

Your love mattered.
Your presence changed everything.
And what you carried will never be invisible here.

CONTENTS

ACKNOWLEDGMENTS

To the physicians, nurses, CNAs, aides, PTs, OTs, SLPs, activity directors, social workers, dietary staff, housekeeping/maintenance staff, administrators, and every behind-the-scenes warrior who holds the world of dementia care together — often without thanks, recognition, or rest:

This book sees you.
This book honors you.
This book exists because of you.

Your work is invisible to many,
but life-changing to the people you serve.

You are the heartbeat of long-term care,
the quiet advocates,
the tired hands,
the strength behind the scenes.

And you deserve a hell of a lot more credit than you get.

AUTHOR'S NOTE

I didn't write this book because dementia is interesting.
I wrote this book because dementia is one of the loneliest experiences in the world.

Not just for the person living it — but for the person caring for them.
The caregiver.
The family member.
The one who "stepped up."
The one who didn't get to opt out.

I've been in the room with hundreds of families.
I've watched the way dementia sneaks in and rearranges a life.
I've seen it strip down identities, rewrite personalities, test marriages, change family dynamics, and break open people in ways they didn't think were possible.

I've also seen — over and over — how love keeps showing up anyway.
Exhausted love.
Frustrated love.

Confused love.
Stubborn love.
Borderline feral survival mode love.
But love, still.

That's why this book exists.

Because caregivers deserve a guide that doesn't sugarcoat anything.
A guide that doesn't talk down to them.
A guide that doesn't pretend dementia is "manageable with a few simple steps."
A guide that doesn't ask them to be saints.
A guide that acknowledges the humor, the heartbreak, the mess, the science, the humanity, the dark nights, the absurd moments, and the grief that begins long before anyone dies.

Caregivers deserve the truth — the clinical truth and the emotional truth.
And they deserve someone to say the thing they carry secretly:

This is hard.
This is complicated.
This is not your fault.

And you're doing better than you think.

I wrote this book for you — the person who showed up even when you were tired, resentful, scared, numb, or burned out.
For you — the person who wants to do the right thing, even when the right thing feels like a moving target.
For you — the caregiver who didn't ask for this job, but did it anyway.

To the families who trusted me with their stories: thank you.
To the caregivers who let me into their hardest moments: thank you.
To every person touched by dementia, in any capacity: this book is my hand on your shoulder.

If you walk away from this book with only one message, let it be this:

You are not alone.
You were never meant to do this alone.
And you don't have to carry the rest of the journey alone either.

Thank you for reading.

Thank you for caring.
Thank you for surviving something that no one can fully understand unless they've lived it.

I f'n hate dementia — but people like you who show up through the confusion, the anger, the grief, and the chaos are the reason humanity still stands a f'n chance.

— Ashley Ivy,
SLP and fellow human who refuses to let caregivers walk through dementia in the dark.

INTRODUCTION
WELCOME TO THE MOST F'D UP CLUB YOU NEVER ASKED TO JOIN

If you're reading this, you've already been hit with something heavy.

A diagnosis.
A decline you can't unsee.
A moment where you realized the person you love is slipping — slowly, quietly, or all at once.

This book won't dilute it:
Dementia is brutal.
It's unfair.
It's relentless.
And it changes everything.

But here's the thing people don't say out loud:

You can learn to navigate this.
You can stay connected.
You can make their world safer, calmer, and easier to understand.
You can survive this — and even find moments of

joy inside the chaos.

This book is half education, half therapy, half "here's how to not lose your sh*t," and half "you've got this."

Yes, I know that's too many halves.
That's what dementia does:
Math stops making sense.
Rules stop applying.
Life becomes a shapeshifter.

So let's get into the truth of it — clinical, practical, no BS.

Welcome to the book that tells it like it is.

PART 1
WHAT THE HELL IS
DEMENTIA ANYWAY?

Most people don't get a real explanation of dementia.

They get pamphlets.

They get vague reassurances.

They get clinical language that explains nothing about what life is actually about to feel like.

This section exists to ground you.

Not with medical jargon.

With honest, human explanations of what dementia is, what it isn't, and why it behaves the way it does.

CHAPTER 1
SO... WHAT THE HELL IS DEMENTIA?

Here's the textbook definition of dementia:

A chronic or progressive syndrome caused by deterioration in memory, thinking, behavior, and the ability to perform everyday activities. Dementia results from various diseases and injuries that affect the brain.

Now that we've gotten the official definition out of the way, let me say what everyone who's ever loved someone with dementia already knows:

STFU.

That definition doesn't help a family who is exhausted, terrified, confused, and trying to understand why the person they love is slipping away in ways that do not fit neatly into a sentence meant for a medical exam.

Real-world dementia isn't a tidy paragraph.
It's a messy, heartbreaking unraveling.
It's a set of daily challenges that don't fit into clinical language.

It's behavior that looks intentional even when it isn't.

It's grief layered on top of more grief.

Dementia isn't normal aging.

Dementia isn't forgetfulness.

Dementia isn't someone being stubborn or "difficult."

Dementia is a brain disease that steals abilities, memories, logic, and orientation one piece at a time.

And this book exists because families deserve someone to finally explain dementia in words real humans understand.

CHAPTER 2
PICTURE THIS

If you really want to understand dementia, you need a visual:

The brain is a long strand of Christmas lights.

Each bulb is something important.
A memory.
A skill.
A habit.
A name.
A movement.
A word.
A personality trait.

At first, one bulb flickers.
Then another.
Then a cluster goes dim.
Then an entire section shuts off.
Some lights blink on and off unpredictably.
Some never come back again.

It isn't because the person isn't trying.
It isn't because they're stubborn.

It isn't because they "don't care."

The wiring is failing.

That's why sometimes you see flashes of clarity in a sea of confusion.
That's why they might remember something vividly one moment and forget it entirely the next.
That's why behaviors shift suddenly.
That's why logic disappears.
That's why repetition happens.
That's why the disease feels unpredictable and chaotic.

The lights are going out, one circuit at a time.

And as heartbreaking as that is, understanding it helps you stop taking the behaviors personally.

CHAPTER 3
THE SIX MOST COMMON TYPES OF DEMENTIA (OR, AS I LIKE TO CALL IT: "WAIT, THERE'S MORE THAN ONE KIND OF HELL?")

Well, Karen, yes.

There is.

Dementia is an umbrella term.

The same way "cancer" is an umbrella term.

Or "car problems" is an umbrella term.

If your mechanic says you have "car problems," you'd say, "No shit, but which ones? My tires? My engine? The little spinny thing I can't pronounce?"

Dementia works the same way.

Different underlying diseases.

Different patterns.

Different symptoms.

Different challenges.

Here are the six types you'll hear about most often.

ALZHEIMER'S DISEASE

The One Everyone Thinks They Understand — and Usually Doesn't

Alzheimer's disease is the most common form of dementia, which is why it's also the most misunderstood. When people hear "Alzheimer's," they picture simple forgetfulness — misplaced keys, repeated questions, a name slipping away.

That's not the full picture.

Not even close.

Alzheimer's is a progressive neurodegenerative disease that slowly destroys the brain's ability to store, retrieve, organize, and use information. Memory is often the first casualty, but it is far from the last.

This disease doesn't just steal memories.
It steals judgment, insight, language, sequencing, emotional regulation, and eventually physical function.

What Families Actually Notice First

Families rarely walk in saying, "We think it's Alzheimer's."

They walk in saying things like:
"She keeps asking the same thing over and over."
"He swears we already talked about this."
"She's different. I can't explain it."
"He gets irritated so fast now."
"She used to handle everything — now she's overwhelmed by nothing."

Early Alzheimer's often shows up as:

- Repeating stories or questions within minutes

- Difficulty following conversations

- Trouble with planning or organizing

- Increased irritability or defensiveness

- Subtle personality changes

- Losing confidence without knowing why

- Anxiety in unfamiliar situations

- Withdrawing socially to avoid embarrassment

The person often knows something is wrong, which makes this stage especially painful. They may try to cover it. Joke it away. Argue. Get defensive. Pretend they "just didn't care anyway."

This isn't denial.
This is fear.

Common Misconceptions That Hurt Families

Misconception #1: "It's just memory loss."

Memory loss is the opening act, not the whole show.
Alzheimer's also affects:

- reasoning

- problem-solving

- emotional control

- decision-making

- insight

Misconception #2: "If you remind them, they'll remember."

Alzheimer's doesn't block access to memories — it damages the ability to store them. You're not dealing with forgetfulness. You're dealing with a filing system that's breaking.

Misconception #3: "They're being difficult."

Resistance, repetition, agitation, and denial are not personality flaws. They're symptoms of a brain losing function.

Misconception #4: "They're still early, so they're fine."

Early Alzheimer's can be emotionally devastating even when daily function looks "okay." The invisible losses hurt just as much as the visible ones.

What Alzheimer's Means for Caregivers — The Part No One Prepares You For

Caring for someone with Alzheimer's is not about reminding harder or explaining better. It's about adjusting expectations — over and over again.

Caregivers often struggle because:

- logic no longer works the way it used to

- reassurance has to replace reasoning

- patience gets tested daily

- grief begins early and lingers

- roles reverse quietly and painfully

As the disease progresses, caregivers must adapt to:

- increased supervision

- repeated conversations

- emotional volatility

- safety concerns

- loss of independence

- increasing physical care needs

The hardest truth?
Love does not stop the disease.
But love does shape how someone experiences it.

Alzheimer's caregiving requires:

- flexibility over control

- reassurance over correction

- presence over perfection

- rest before collapse

You are not failing if this feels hard.
It is hard.
By design.

VASCULAR DEMENTIA

The One That Comes in Drops, Not a Straight Line

Vascular dementia is the second most common form of dementia — and one of the most confusing for families.
That's because it doesn't follow a smooth, predictable decline.
It doesn't fade gently.
It drops.

Vascular dementia is caused by reduced blood flow to the brain, often due to strokes, mini-strokes (TIAs), heart disease, uncontrolled blood pressure, diabetes, or vascular damage over time. When the brain doesn't get enough oxygen, brain tissue dies. And once it dies, it doesn't regenerate.

This is not a memory problem first.
This is a blood flow problem that becomes a brain problem.

What Families Actually Notice First

Families often describe vascular dementia like this:
"He was fine… then suddenly he wasn't."
"She declined overnight."
"He took a big step backward and never recovered."
"She has good days and then awful ones."
"Every time something medical happens, he gets worse."

Unlike Alzheimer's, vascular dementia often looks like:

- sudden changes after a stroke or hospitalization

- noticeable drops in function instead of gradual decline

- slowed thinking and processing

- trouble with attention and focus

- difficulty planning or problem-solving

- emotional changes, including depression or apathy

- physical changes like weakness, balance issues, or gait changes

One of the hallmark features is what caregivers describe as "stair-step decline."

They'll stabilize for a while.
Then something happens.
And they drop.

And they don't bounce back.

The Stair-Step Reality —
Why This Feels So Jarring

With vascular dementia, caregivers are often caught off guard because:

- recovery is expected after illness or stroke

- rehab looks promising at first

- the person seems "mostly themselves"

- hope keeps sneaking back in

But vascular damage accumulates.

Each stroke, infection, fall, surgery, or medical event can:

- worsen cognition

- increase confusion

- reduce mobility

- amplify behavioral changes

This is why families often feel like they're living in a cycle of false hope followed by grief.

Common Misconceptions That Make It Harder

Misconception #1: "They'll improve with therapy."

Therapy can help maximize function — but it cannot restore dead brain tissue.

Misconception #2: "They seem okay most of the time."

Vascular dementia often hides in plain sight. Slower thinking, poor judgment, and impaired decision-making are easily mistaken for laziness, stubbornness, or personality changes.

Misconception #3: "If we manage the medical issues, the dementia will stop."

Managing risk factors can slow progression, but it does not erase existing damage.

What Vascular Dementia Means for Caregivers

Caregivers of someone with vascular dementia often feel emotionally whiplashed.

One day:
"They're doing better!"

The next:
"What just happened?"

Caregivers must prepare for:

- unpredictable declines

- increased physical care needs earlier

- combined cognitive and mobility challenges

- higher fall risk

- emotional changes like apathy or depression

- safety concerns related to poor judgment

This type of dementia demands constant adjustment — not because you're doing something wrong, but because the disease does not move in straight lines.

The Emotional Toll — Again... No One Talks About This Part

Vascular dementia steals confidence quickly — both from the person living with it and from the caregiver trying to keep up.

Caregivers often say:
"I don't trust leaving them alone anymore."
"I never know what version I'm getting."
"I'm always bracing for the next drop."

"I feel like I'm waiting for the next shoe to fall."

That feeling?
That's not anxiety.
That's lived experience.

What Helps — Even When You Can't Fix It

With vascular dementia, the most powerful tools are:

- structure

- routine

- medical management

- realistic expectations

- support for the caregiver

You are not failing if progress feels fragile.
You are navigating a disease built on instability.

LEWY BODY DEMENTIA

When Reality Flickers and the Rules Keep Changing

Lewy Body Dementia (LBD) is one of the most

misunderstood — and most destabilizing —
dementias for families and caregivers.
Not because it's rare.
But because it refuses to follow the rules people
expect dementia to follow.

Lewy Body Dementia is caused by abnormal
protein deposits (Lewy bodies) in the brain. These
deposits disrupt multiple brain systems at once —
thinking, movement, sleep, perception, and
behavior.

That's why LBD doesn't feel like "just memory
loss."
It feels like cognitive chaos.

What Families Actually Notice First

Families often say things like:
"Some days he's completely normal."
"She'll have full conversations… then be gone the
next hour."
"He sees things that aren't there — and they feel
real to him."
"Doctors keep changing the diagnosis."
"I feel like I'm losing my mind trying to keep up."

Early signs often include:

- vivid visual hallucinations (people, animals, children, bugs)

- extreme fluctuations in attention and alertness

- episodes of confusion followed by startling clarity

- REM sleep behavior disorder (acting out dreams)

- slowed movement, stiffness, tremors, shuffling gait

- sensitivity to medications (especially antipsychotics)

This dementia shape-shifts — and that unpredictability is what breaks caregivers.

The Hallucinations —
The Part That Terrifies Families

Hallucinations in Lewy Body Dementia are not subtle.
They are not fleeting.

They are not "just confusion."

They are often:

- detailed

- recurring

- emotionally charged

- fully believed

People with LBD may:

- talk to people who aren't there

- insist strangers are in the house

- accuse caregivers of hiding people

- react with fear, anger, or defensiveness

Correcting them usually makes things worse.

Because to them —
the hallucination is real.

And trying to logic someone out of a neurological experience only escalates distress.

The Fluctuations —
Why This Dementia Gaslights Everyone

One of the cruelest aspects of Lewy Body Dementia is the dramatic fluctuation in cognition.

A person may:

- be fully oriented in the morning

- confused and agitated by afternoon

- completely lucid again at dinner

This leads families to think:
"They're doing better!"
"Maybe it's not dementia."
"They were fine yesterday."/And then —
everything collapses again.

This back-and-forth creates false hope, delayed diagnosis, and immense emotional exhaustion for caregivers.

Movement Changes —
Why It Gets Confused With Parkinson's

Lewy Body Dementia shares symptoms with Parkinson's disease:

- rigidity

- tremors

- slowed movements

- balance issues

- falls

Sometimes dementia symptoms appear first.
Sometimes movement symptoms appear first.
Sometimes both show up together.

This overlap often leads to:

- misdiagnosis

- delayed support

- medication complications

Medication Sensitivity —
This Part Is Dangerous

People with Lewy Body Dementia can have severe
reactions to common antipsychotic medications.

Reactions may include:

- extreme sedation

- sudden cognitive collapse

- increased confusion

- worsening movement symptoms

- life-threatening responses

This is why accurate diagnosis matters.
And why caregivers must advocate fiercely.

What Lewy Body Dementia Means for Caregivers

Caregivers of someone with LBD live in a constant state of adjustment.

You're managing:

- hallucinations

- movement issues

- sleep disturbances

- sudden confusion

- moments of stunning clarity

- emotional volatility

- safety concerns

- medication risks

And you're doing it without predictability.

This is not a "routine-friendly" dementia.
This is a brace-yourself dementia.

The Emotional Toll —
This One Hits Differently

Caregivers often say:
"I never know what's coming."
"I don't trust the calm."
"The good moments make the bad ones hurt more."
"I feel like I'm grieving over and over."

That's because Lewy Body Dementia gives you just enough clarity to remind you who they were — and then takes it away again.

What Actually Helps

With LBD, the most effective approaches include:

- validating emotions instead of correcting facts

- simplifying the environment

- keeping lighting consistent

- reducing visual clutter

- managing sleep carefully

- working with neurologists who understand LBD

- building caregiver support early

And most importantly:

- believing caregivers when they say something feels off.

Because with Lewy Body Dementia — it usually is.

FRONTOTEMPORAL DEMENTIA

When Personality Goes First and Memory Lags Behind

Frontotemporal Dementia (FTD) is often the most

shocking dementia for families — not because of memory loss, but because the person changes before anyone understands why.

FTD affects the frontal and temporal lobes of the brain — the areas responsible for:

- personality

- judgment

- impulse control

- social behavior

- emotional regulation

- language

That means this dementia doesn't start with forgetting.
It starts with being different.

What Families Actually Notice First

Families often say:
"This isn't like them at all."
"They've become rude, blunt, or inappropriate."
"They don't seem to care anymore."

"They say things they never would have said."
"They've lost their filter."
"They've become impulsive or reckless."
"They're not sad about it — I am."

Early signs often include:

- personality changes

- loss of empathy

- inappropriate jokes or comments

- impulsive spending

- poor judgment

- emotional flatness

- social withdrawal

- rigid routines or obsessions

- overeating or food fixation

- apathy without obvious sadness

Memory may still be surprisingly intact early on.
Which makes this dementia easy to misinterpret.

The Misdiagnosis Problem —
Why Families Feel Crazy

FTD is frequently misdiagnosed as:

- depression

- anxiety

- midlife crisis

- bipolar disorder

- substance abuse

- personality disorder

- marital issues

Why?

Because on paper, the person can still:

- remember names

- recall facts

- perform tasks

- hold conversations

But emotionally?

Socially?

Behaviorally?

They are not the same person.

This leads families to:

- argue more

- feel blamed

- feel dismissed

- feel like they're "overreacting"

You're not.

Behavior Changes — The Hardest Part

In FTD, behavior changes are neurological, not intentional.

This can include:

- saying offensive things without remorse

- touching people inappropriately

- violating social norms

- making unsafe decisions

- showing no insight into consequences

- becoming emotionally cold or indifferent

This is devastating for spouses and adult children. Because the person looks "fine" — but acts unrecognizable.

Loss of Empathy — Why It Feels So Personal

One of the most painful features of FTD is loss of empathy.

They may:

- stop asking how you are

- not comfort you when you cry

- seem indifferent to major events

- fail to recognize emotional cues

Families often interpret this as:

- selfishness

- narcissism

- cruelty

- lack of love

But it's none of those.
The emotional processing centers are failing.

Language Variants —
When Words Fall Apart

Some forms of FTD primarily affect language.

People may:

- struggle to find words

- lose vocabulary

- misuse words

- stop understanding language

- become silent over time

This can happen without memory loss, which is deeply confusing for families.

Why This Dementia Breaks Families — The One That Continuously Makes Me Clutch My Chest

FTD often hits younger adults — sometimes in their 40s, 50s, or early 60s.

That means:

- careers are interrupted

- children are still at home

- finances are impacted

- marriages are strained

- expectations are shattered

Caregivers are often spouses who never expected to become one this early.

This is not the dementia people prepare for.
This is the dementia that upends lives midstream.

What Helps (and What Doesn't)

What doesn't help:

- reasoning

- consequences

- shame

- lectures

- "They know better"

What helps:

- structure

- consistency

- environmental controls

- supervision

- external boundaries

- professional support

- caregiver education

Because in FTD:
Internal brakes are gone.
External support becomes essential.

What Caregivers Need to Hear

"You did not cause this."

"You cannot reason it away."
"You are not failing."
"You are not imagining things."
"You are not heartless for grieving who they used to be."

FTD steals personality before memory.
And that grief is brutal.

The Bottom Line

Frontotemporal Dementia is not about forgetting.
It's about becoming someone else neurologically.

And caregivers are left loving a body that no longer holds the person they knew — while the world expects them to "be patient" with behavior no one understands.

You are not alone in this.
And what you're experiencing is real.

MIXED DEMENTIA

When Dementia Flips You Off and Refuses to Follow One Set of Rules

Mixed Dementia is exactly what it sounds like —

more than one type of dementia happening at the same time.

And it is far more common than most families realize.

The most frequent combination is:

- Alzheimer's disease + Vascular dementia

But it can also include:

- Alzheimer's + Lewy Body dementia

- Alzheimer's + Parkinson's disease dementia

- Vascular dementia + another neurodegenerative condition

Which means the brain is being hit from multiple angles at once.

Why Mixed Dementia Is So Confusing

Families often say:
"Some days are good. Some days are terrifying."
"The decline isn't steady — it jumps."
"They remember things sometimes but not others."

"The symptoms don't match what the doctor told us."
"Nothing about this feels predictable."

That's because it isn't.

Mixed dementia doesn't follow a clean timeline.
It doesn't stick to one symptom pattern.
It doesn't respect stages.

It pulls features from different diseases and blends them into one unpredictable experience.

What Families Actually Notice First

You may see:

- memory loss that looks like Alzheimer's

- sudden declines that look like vascular dementia

- fluctuations in clarity

- mood changes

- confusion that worsens after illness or stress

- behavior changes that don't quite fit one diagnosis

- uneven skill loss (some abilities intact, others gone)

One day they can:
balance a checkbook,
recall old memories,
hold a conversation.

And the next day they:
can't follow a simple instruction,
forget where they are,
become agitated or withdrawn.

Families often feel like they're losing their footing because there's no consistent rulebook.

The Step-Down Pattern —
Why It Feels Like Free-Fall

In mixed dementia, decline often happens in steps, not slopes.

Things may look stable for weeks or months.
Then a sudden drop.

Common triggers:

- infections (especially UTIs)

- dehydration

- hospitalization

- anesthesia

- medication changes

- strokes or mini-strokes

- emotional stress

After each drop, some abilities may return. Some won't.

This creates false hope followed by fresh grief — over and over.

Why Caregiving Feels So Hard

Caregivers struggle with mixed dementia because:

- strategies that worked last week stop working

- behaviors change without warning

- symptoms contradict each other

- doctors give vague answers

- progression feels chaotic

You're not doing anything wrong.
The disease itself is inconsistent.

Medical Reality —
Why Diagnosis Often Comes Late

Mixed dementia is oftentimes only truly confirmed after death - through brain examination.

During life, doctors may say:
"Probable Alzheimer's"
"Likely vascular components"
"Cognitive decline with mixed features"

This uncertainty leaves families desperate for clarity.

But here's the truth:
Your lived experience matters more than the label.

What Helps in Mixed Dementia

Because the brain is failing in multiple systems, care must be:

- flexible

- observant

- responsive

- forgiving

Helpful approaches include:

- consistent routines

- hydration and nutrition monitoring

- medication reviews

- infection prevention

- minimizing hospitalizations

- calm environments

- caregiver education

- realistic expectations

And above all:

- adjusting care to the worst day, not the best one

Because best days lie.
Worst days tell the truth.

Emotional Toll on Caregivers

Mixed dementia creates a unique kind of grief:
hope followed by loss,
clarity followed by confusion,
progress followed by regression.

It's exhausting.
It's destabilizing.
It makes you question your judgment.

You are not weak for feeling worn down.
This disease is relentless.

The Bottom Line

Mixed dementia is not "milder."
It's not "a little of this, a little of that."

It is compound damage to a fragile system.

And caregivers deserve honesty:
This form of dementia is harder to predict, harder
to manage, and harder to emotionally survive.

If this is your reality — you are not alone.

And nothing about this confusion means you're failing.

PARKINSON'S DISEASE DEMENTIA

When Movement Fails First — and Thinking Follows

Parkinson's Disease Dementia (PDD) is different from many other dementias because the movement disorder comes first.

The person is diagnosed with Parkinson's disease — sometimes years earlier — and dementia develops later as the disease spreads deeper into the brain.

This distinction matters.

If dementia appears before or at the same time as movement symptoms, it's more likely Lewy Body Dementia.
If Parkinson's comes first and cognition declines later, it's Parkinson's Disease Dementia.

The symptoms may look similar.
The timeline is the key difference.

What Families Notice First

Families often don't realize dementia is developing because Parkinson's already explains so much.

They think:
"That's just the Parkinson's."
"They're slow because of stiffness."
"They're tired because movement takes effort."
"They're quiet because talking is hard."

But gradually, cognitive changes emerge that can't be explained by movement alone.

Early signs often include:

- slowed thinking (bradyphrenia)

- difficulty planning or organizing

- trouble multitasking

- reduced problem-solving ability

- word-finding pauses

- impaired attention

- decreased facial expression (often mistaken

for emotional withdrawal)

The person may seem mentally "foggy" or delayed — not forgetful at first, but slowed.

How It Progresses

As Parkinson's Disease Dementia advances, families may notice:

- memory impairment

- visual hallucinations

- delusions or paranoia

- confusion that worsens in the evening

- difficulty following conversations

- impaired judgment

- emotional flatness or sudden mood shifts

Hallucinations are common and often involve:

- people

- animals

- shadows or movement at the edges of

vision

Unlike psychosis, these hallucinations may feel very real but are not always distressing — until they are.

The Role of Medications —
Why Things Can Suddenly Change

Parkinson's medications walk a dangerous line.

They help movement.
But they can worsen:

- hallucinations

- confusion

- agitation

- impulsivity

Medication changes can cause sudden cognitive crashes or behavioral changes, which terrifies families.

You didn't "miss something."
The brain chemistry is delicate — and reactive.

Why Caregiving Is So Physically Demanding

Parkinson's Disease Dementia doesn't just affect thinking — it locks the body in place.

Caregivers often manage:

- freezing episodes

- falls

- rigidity

- shuffling gait

- swallowing difficulties

- drooling

- masked facial expression

- fatigue

At the same time, cognition declines.

This combination makes caregiving physically AND mentally exhausting.

Communication Challenges

Speech changes can include:

- soft voice

- monotone speech

- reduced initiation

- delayed responses

- difficulty expressing needs

Caregivers may assume the person is disengaged or uninterested.

They aren't.
Their brain and body are simply struggling to keep up.

Emotional Changes Families See

Families often describe:

- apathy

- anxiety

- depression

- emotional blunting

- sudden irritability

These changes are neurological — not a loss of love or interest.

The Hidden Grief

Parkinson's Disease Dementia carries a unique grief because:

- the decline feels like betrayal after years of fighting Parkinson's

- families feel blindsided

- expectations were set around movement, not cognition

You thought you understood the disease.
Then it changed the rules.

What Helps

Helpful strategies include:

- simplifying choices

- allowing extra processing time

- maintaining predictable routines

- minimizing environmental clutter

- using calm, direct communication

- monitoring medication effects closely

- involving movement and speech specialists early

And most importantly:

- slowing down your expectations

The brain needs more time.
So does the body.

The Bottom Line

Parkinson's Disease Dementia is not "just Parkinson's getting worse."

It is a new phase of the disease that affects identity, communication, reasoning, and independence.

Caregivers are often unprepared for this shift — and that lack of preparation causes unnecessary suffering.

If this is the road you're on:
Your confusion makes sense.
Your exhaustion is valid.

Your grief is real.

And you are not failing.

CHAPTER 4
WHAT DEMENTIA IS NOT

Dementia is not stubbornness.

Dementia is not laziness.

Dementia is not bad manners.

Dementia is not someone "acting out."

Dementia is not an attitude problem.

Dementia is not someone "not trying hard enough."

Dementia is not intentional.

Dementia is a disease disrupting the way the brain sends, receives, organizes, and processes information.

Dementia is a disease that changes the brain, which means the behaviors you see are neurological, not personal.

Let me say that again for the ones in the back:

Dementia is a disease that changes the brain, which means the behaviors you see are neurological, NOT personal.

CHAPTER 5
WHEN SOMETHING FEELS OFF (BUT NO ONE HAS A NAME FOR IT)

Dementia rarely kicks the door in.
It sneaks in quietly, through cracks you barely notice.

Overall, here's what loved ones usually see first:

- Repeating stories.

- Misplacing everyday items.

- Forgetting recent conversations.

- Losing track of dates, appointments, or time.

- Getting overwhelmed by tasks that were previously simple.

- Mood swings.

- Changes in sleep.

- Withdrawing socially.

- Confusion in unfamiliar places.

- Difficulty following conversations.

- Trouble managing money or bills.

- Starting tasks but never finishing them.

- Saying "What?" more often.

- Increasing irritability or defensiveness.

- Increased anxiety or fear when routines change.

Most families don't connect these dots right away because none of these alone scream dementia. But together, they paint the beginning of the picture.

CHAPTER 6
WHY DEMENTIA BEHAVES
THE WAY IT DOES

Spoiler alert: dementia doesn't give a damn who you are.

It doesn't care if you have a PhD, walked on the moon, ran a successful business, raised five kids, or went viral on Instagram.

It doesn't care if you saved Old Man Johnny's cat from a tree in 1987.

It behaves the same way because the disease attacks the wiring of the brain, not the résumé of the person living in it.

Every dementia behavior traces back to a single truth:

The brain has lost access to information that used to be automatic.

Memory loss creates repetition.

Fear creates agitation.

Confusion creates anger.

Disorientation creates wandering.

Loss of sequencing creates difficulty with tasks.

Loss of inhibition creates inappropriate comments.
Loss of judgment creates unsafe decisions.
Loss of time sense creates nighttime confusion.
Loss of language pathways creates frustration and emotional outbursts.

None of it is random.
None of it is spiteful.
None of it is personal.

It's the wiring failing.
It's the Christmas lights going out.

And now that you understand the "why," you're ready for Part Two:
the stages of dementia, explained in real human language.

FROM THE FIELD: HIDE YO KIDS, HIDE YO WIFE

Let me drop in one of those moments that perfectly captures how dementia can turn your day upside down, crack you up, humble you, and remind you that flexibility is not a skill — it's a survival mechanism.

It was one of those days at work.
The kind where every staff member is whispering, "There must be a full moon," even though none of us have checked an actual calendar.

Agitation up.
Sleep down.
Everyone pacing, yelling, crying, or needing something urgent in the same ten minutes.

I was walking down the hall, exhausted and mentally fried, trying to breathe before going into the next room.

And for whatever reason — maybe brain fog, maybe divine intervention — the viral meme

popped into my head:
"Hide yo kids, hide yo wife…"

So I muttered it under my breath while walking.

Not loudly.
Not intentionally.
Just clinician brain on fumes.

And then I heard a voice behind me —
one of my residents with dementia, following me
quietly —
say:

"Okay, come on honey… where we hidin'?"

I stopped dead in the hallway.

What do you even do with that?

So I pivoted — clinician mode + improv comedy
mode — and said:

"I guess right over here! We're playing hide and
seek and I bet we win. They ain't got nothin' on
us."

And this person, bless them, nodded like we'd
rehearsed the whole thing.

Just like that, we were teammates.
Partners in crime.
Co-champions of a game I didn't mean to start.
Hiding behind the nurses' station like fugitives.

And that's the thing:

Dementia demands flexibility you didn't know you
had.

You can't control the moment —
but you can roll with it.
You can redirect with a smile.
You can turn confusion into connection.

The relief on their face?
Pure gold.

Because in that moment,
we weren't dealing with confusion or fear
or the weight of cognitive decline.

We were just two humans
having a ridiculous hallway adventure
in the middle of a chaos-filled day.

That's dementia.
Not always tragic.

Not always dramatic.
Sometimes just beautifully absurd.

These are the moments that get you through the
hard ones.
These are the moments that remind you
the person is still in there —
just in different flashes,
in different ways,
at different times.

Sometimes the best therapeutic approach
isn't a perfectly structured technique.

Sometimes it's just saying:
"Alright, I guess we're hiding now."

PART 2
THE STAGES OF DEMENTIA

The stages of dementia aren't neat.
They don't follow a straight line.
And they don't look exactly the same for every person.

But understanding the general progression gives you something powerful:
context.

This section explains the stages of dementia in real-world language — not to predict every moment, but to help you recognize patterns, prepare emotionally, and stop feeling blindsided by what's coming.

Before We Break This Down

If you've been looking for a clean, predictable timeline for dementia, I need to say this up front: There isn't one.
The stages you're about to read are not neat boxes.
They don't arrive on schedule.
They don't progress politely.
People don't move through them at the same pace, and they don't experience them in the same way.
Some stages overlap.
Some show up out of order.
Some linger far longer than expected.
Others seem to arrive overnight.

The purpose of these stages is not to label your person or to predict an exact future.
The purpose is orientation.

To help you recognize what you're seeing.
To help you understand why behaviors are changing.
To help you stop blaming yourself, them, or the relationship.
To help you prepare — emotionally, practically, and medically — for what may come next.

Families often ask,
"Which stage are we in?"

A better question is often,
"Which abilities are slipping — and which ones are
still intact?"

Dementia is not a straight line.
It's a slow erosion with unpredictable edges.

You may recognize pieces of multiple stages at
once.
That doesn't mean you're misunderstanding the
disease.
It means you're seeing it accurately.

Read these stages as a map, not a verdict.
A way to make sense of what feels chaotic.
A way to name what you're living.
A way to remember that none of this is random —
even when it feels unbearable.

And, most importantly:
These stages describe the disease.

They do not define the person.
They do not erase the love.

They do not cancel the moments of connection that still matter.

With all of that in mind, let's walk through them — together.

CHAPTER 7
STAGE 1:
THE SUBTLE SHIFT

The earliest stage of dementia is the most confusing because everything feels "off," but nothing feels serious.

You might notice small slips that come and go, a weird hesitancy, a moment of blankness that lingers too long.

They may ask a question twice.

They may search for a word that used to be automatic.

They may miss a detail in a simple story.

Nothing big enough to sound the alarm.

Everything big enough to make you pause.

Stage 1 is where families say, "Well... everyone forgets things sometimes."

And that's true.

Everyone does.

But dementia-level forgetting has a different flavor.

It's stickier.

It's heavier.

It comes with a different look in the eyes.

A moment where they're suddenly... not anchored.

In Stage 1, you begin grieving quietly, even if you don't realize that's what's happening. Something deep inside you knows a page has turned.
In this stage, people often compensate well.
They use notes, jokes, deflection, or avoidance to cover the gaps.
They may laugh off mistakes or blame stress, aging, or being "too busy."
Many still function independently, which makes loved ones question their own instincts.

This is also the stage where caregivers doubt themselves the most.
You may feel uneasy but unable to explain why.
Trust that instinct.
Dementia often announces itself not with obvious loss, but with a quiet sense that something is no longer lining up the way it used to.

CAREGIVER REALITY CHECK — STAGE 1

If you feel unsettled but can't explain why, you're not imagining it.

Early dementia rarely announces itself loudly.

It whispers.

You are allowed to notice patterns before you have proof.

You are allowed to trust your gut even when others dismiss it.

Early awareness is not overreacting — it's information.

CHAPTER 8
STAGE 2:
THE CRACKS IN THE
FOUNDATION

This is where you can feel a shift in the ground beneath you.

The cracks widen.

The gaps become noticeable.

They start losing their place in conversations.

They may forget to pay a bill, forget an appointment, forget where they put something important.

They might become anxious in situations that never bothered them before.

They might withdraw because the world suddenly feels too fast and too loud.

They might avoid social situations because conversation feels exhausting or embarrassing.

In Stage 2, logic starts slipping.

Multi-step tasks begin to overwhelm them.

Patterns shift.

Their confidence begins to erode because they can feel something happening but can't articulate it.

The fear is real, but so is the determination.

They'll try to cover the cracks, patch the holes, hide the confusion.

But you see it.

You feel it.

Even if no one else does yet.

Stage 2 is the stage where families start having private whispers: Is this… dementia? Should we say something?

Should we wait?

It's the stage where denial becomes a warm blanket no one wants to put down.

As the cracks widen, effort increases.

The brain works harder to do what once came easily, and that effort shows up as fatigue, irritability, or withdrawal.

This is often when loved ones begin stepping in "just a little" — helping with reminders, checking behind tasks, double-confirming details.

The shift into caregiving has usually already begun, even if no one is calling it that yet.

CAREGIVER REALITY CHECK — STAGE 2

This is often where caregiving quietly begins — without a name, a plan, or support.
Helping "just a little" still counts as caregiving.
Feeling worried does not mean you're negative.
Not knowing what to do yet does not mean you're failing.

You are adjusting to a moving target — give yourself grace.

CHAPTER 9
STAGE 3:
THE DISAPPEARING MIDDLE
GROUND

Stage 3 is where the world begins to divide into two categories:

things they can still do quickly and things they suddenly cannot do at all.

There is less middle ground, less predictability, less consistency.

You may notice them losing the ability to track time.

They may get lost in familiar places.

They might tell the same story three times in thirty minutes.

Tasks that used to take five minutes now take twenty.

Tasks that used to take twenty minutes are suddenly impossible.

This is also the stage where emotional changes hit harder.

Irritability.

Anxiety.

Suspicion.

Frustration.

They know something is wrong, and that awareness burns.

Their brain is working harder to compensate, and the strain shows.

Caregivers may find themselves walking on eggshells — trying to help without triggering fear or humiliation.

This is where learning new communication strategies becomes essential.

How you say things matters more than what you say.

CAREGIVER REALITY CHECK — STAGE 3

If your loved one seems more irritable, defensive, or emotional, it's not because they're becoming difficult.

It's because they still know something is wrong — and that awareness hurts.

You are not required to fix the fear.
You are not required to win arguments.

Your job is safety, reassurance, and connection —
not logic.

CHAPTER 10
STAGE 4:
WHEN THE WORLD STARTS WARPING

Stage 4 is where dementia becomes undeniable.

Not just to you — but to everyone.

The person loses the ability to hide what's happening.

Conversations fall apart.

Planning is gone.

Judgment is impaired.

They may forget major life events.

They may forget parts of their personal history.

They may confuse timelines.

They may struggle with basic reasoning.

They may become lost in places they've lived for years.

This is also the stage where time becomes slippery.

Days blend.

Seasons blur.

The brain cannot organize information efficiently anymore, and everything becomes overwhelming.

Stage 4 is heartbreaking because the person still has moments of clarity, humor, and personality — but those moments are surrounded by longer stretches of fog.
It feels like watching someone fade in and out of the present.

This is the stage where families must stop doing things "as they've always been done."
You cannot reason someone out of confusion.
You cannot correct someone into clarity.
You cannot push a brain to function beyond its ability.

This stage requires compassion, patience, and a total reframing of how you communicate.
By this point, the disease is interfering with reasoning, sequencing, and judgment in ways that cannot be hidden.
Safety becomes a real concern.
Independence starts slipping in meaningful ways, even if the person insists they are "fine."

Families often experience grief and conflict here — grief for what's being lost, and conflict over what to do next.

This stage forces hard conversations about driving, living arrangements, and increased supervision. Avoidance makes this stage harder, not easier.

CAREGIVER REALITY CHECK — STAGE 4

This stage forces decisions families often avoid — and avoiding them makes everything harder.

Again, you cannot reason a damaged brain into clarity.
Correcting confusion usually increases distress.
Support is not surrender.

Hard choices do not mean you love them less — they mean you're facing reality with courage.

CHAPTER 11
STAGE 5:
THE BREAKING POINT
WHERE INDEPENDENCE
ISN'T SAFE

Stage 5 is the point where independence is no
longer realistic or safe.

The person cannot manage medication, finances,
meals, or daily tasks without oversight.

They may forget names of close family members.

They may wander, leaving the house without
understanding where they're going.

They may misread situations and react in ways that
make no sense to anyone around them.

Bathing becomes a battle.

Dressing becomes confusing.

Instructions become overwhelming.

Sundowning increases.

Sleep becomes unpredictable.

Eating becomes inconsistent.

They may accuse you of things you didn't do or
insist something happened that never did.

This is not personality.

This is neurological failure.

Stage 5 is where caregivers begin to break under the weight of constant vigilance.
This is where burnout spikes.
This is where guilt tries to move into your home like a roommate.
It is also the stage where many families realize they need more support.

This stage marks a turning point:
good intentions are no longer enough.
Love alone cannot compensate for neurological decline.
Caregiving becomes constant, and the margin for error shrinks.

Many caregivers reach physical and emotional exhaustion here.
If you're wondering whether you can keep going the same way you have been — that question itself is information.
This is often the stage where outside help is no longer optional; it's protective.
This is not failure.
This is humanity.

CAREGIVER REALITY CHECK — STAGE 5

If you feel like you're breaking, that is not weakness — it is a warning sign.

One person cannot safely do the work of a full care team.
Burnout is not a personal failure — it's a predictable outcome of constant vigilance.

Asking for help is not quitting.
It is protecting everyone involved.

CHAPTER 12
STAGE 6:
WHEN THE BRAIN FORGETS THE BODY

This is where dementia shifts from cognitive decline to whole-body involvement.

They begin forgetting how to move their muscles in sequence.

Walking becomes shuffling.

Balance falters.

Transfers require help.

Toileting becomes increasingly difficult.

Incontinence becomes common.

Swallowing becomes risky.

Sleep overtakes most of the day.

Communication drops to a handful of words, then to sounds, then silence.

The emotional brain still recognizes tone, affection, safety — but language becomes too heavy to carry.

This is a tender stage.

A brutal stage.

A sacred stage.

Caregiving becomes physical, intimate, exhausting work.

Touch replaces words.

Tone replaces logic.

Safety replaces independence.

Emotional connection still exists, but it must be communicated through presence rather than conversation.

And yet somehow, this stage brings some of the gentlest moments of connection — a squeeze of a hand, a small smile, a head leaning toward your voice.

Love becomes quieter, but no less present.

This stage is heavy, but it can also be unexpectedly tender.

Small moments — a calm expression, a familiar song, a hand squeeze — carry enormous weight.

Caregivers often need more support than they realize here, especially to protect their own bodies and health.

CAREGIVER REALITY CHECK — STAGE 6

Love no longer looks like conversation — it looks

like presence.

Even when words are gone, the emotional brain still
feels:
tone,
touch,
safety,
familiarity.

You matter in this stage way more than you realize
— even when it feels invisible.

CHAPTER 13
STAGE 7:
THE FINAL DESCENT

Stage 7 is where the disease overtakes everything.
The person becomes fully dependent on others for
every aspect of care.
They sleep most of the day.
They no longer walk.
They no longer talk.
Swallowing becomes extremely limited.
The body thins.
The muscles tighten.
Breathing shifts.
Moments of awareness become rare and precious.

This stage is not dramatic.
It is slow.
Soft.
Inevitable.

You may feel helpless, terrified, heartbroken,
relieved, guilty for the relief, grateful for the quiet
moments, devastated by the loss of connection.
All of it is normal.

Stage 7 is the final chapter of dementia — the last miles of a long, painful, sacred journey. The end is near, but the love remains fierce.

This stage requires a shift from doing to being.
From fixing to comforting.
From intervention to presence.
The goal is no longer prolonging function, but preserving dignity, comfort, and peace.

Families often need reassurance here — reassurance that what they're seeing is natural, that they haven't caused it, and that love still matters even when responses are minimal.
It does.
Profoundly.

This is where caregiving becomes less about tasks and more about witnessing — holding space for a life completing itself.

CAREGIVER REALITY CHECK — STAGE 7

Nothing you're feeling here is wrong.

Relief does not cancel grief.

Grief does not cancel love.

Exhaustion does not cancel devotion.

You are not witnessing failure — you are witnessing completion.

Your presence still matters, even in silence.

FROM THE FIELD: THE NURSE WHO BECAME MY CHEF... AND STARTED CUSSING

She wasn't a chef. And she didn't cuss — at least not before dementia. But dementia gave her a whole new vocabulary and an even bigger personality.

She was one of those women who could shut a whole room down with one glare. Standoffish. Sharp. Blunt. But with me? She softened. She'd light up. We had our own world.

One of the only ways to get her engaged during those later-stage days was with our running joke.

I'd walk in and say, "Hey girl, you working today?"

She'd snap her head up, eyes suddenly awake, and say, "Yeah, you know I am." And just like that, she'd be alive again — present, connected, laughing.

I'd ask if we should take our lunch break at the same time, and she'd surprise me almost every day with, "Well let's go then. I'm on my break now."

We'd walk to the dining room, and she'd look at the food like she owned the place. In her story — the one dementia helped her build — she was the top-tier chef. And I? I was her cook. Beneath her. Holding the plate. Taking her orders.

And the truth is… I'd take that job any day.

Her family told me she never cussed in her life before the disease. But dementia untucked her filter. She'd tap her leg, look around, and mutter things like, "Well if this ain't some shit," or "You know damn well I'll be here all night cleaning up." It cracked me up every time because it was so opposite of the woman she used to be.

Some days she didn't say anything at all. I'd find her sitting by the window with a curtain bunched in her lap like a blanket. I'd sit next to her in silence — long stretches of silence. She'd look at me every once in a while and smile. A quiet, soft smile that told me she felt safe.

Many times I would be completely finished with my day, keys in hand — headed out the door — but I stayed. And it was my honor. Because peace matters. And she deserved someone to sit in it with her.

This is dementia.
This is love.
This is the work.

PART 3
BEING A CAREGIVER
WITHOUT LOSING
YOURSELF

Caregiving does not come with a manual — and it certainly doesn't come with permission to take care of yourself while you're doing it.

This part of the book exists because too many caregivers disappear quietly while trying to hold someone else together.
Needs pile up.
Sleep disappears.
Guilt gets loud.
And somehow, caring for yourself starts to feel selfish instead of necessary.

This section is not about perfection.
It's about survival.
It's about boundaries, burnout, honesty, and learning how to stay human while doing inhumanly hard work.

You don't have to read this part in order.
You don't have to agree with every word.

But if anything here helps you breathe a little easier, feel a little less alone, or recognize yourself with more compassion — then it's doing exactly what it's meant to do.

CHAPTER 14
THE CAREGIVER SURVIVAL GUIDE

Caregiving is a role that turns ordinary people into exhausted, overextended, fiercely devoted human beings who often forget they are human at all.
The world glorifies caregiving as noble work, but it rarely tells the truth about what it feels like to carry someone else's life on your shoulders while your own life slowly shrinks.

You cannot save someone if you disappear in the process.
You cannot protect someone if your body is shutting down.
You cannot think clearly if you're running on four hours of broken sleep.

You cannot pour from an empty cup, and caregiving has a way of smashing the cup on the ground.

This chapter gives you what no one gives caregivers soon enough: the truth, the tools, and the permission to stop trying to be superhuman.

The Truth You Have to Accept to Survive

You cannot fix dementia.
You cannot reverse it, outsmart it, or talk it out of
happening.
Your job is not to cure.
Your job is to care.

You will lose your patience.
You will snap.
You will cry.
You will wish this wasn't your life.
None of that makes you a bad caregiver.
It makes you human.

They are not doing this on purpose.
The confusion, repetition, fear, agitation,
accusations, wandering, resistance—every part of it
is coming from a brain losing function.
Again, it is neurological, not personal.

Your feelings are valid.
You can love them and still feel resentful.
You can want to protect them and still feel trapped.
You can cry from heartbreak and cry from
frustration in the same hour.

You need breaks.
Not want.
Need.
Your body, brain, and heart cannot withstand the demands of dementia around the clock.

You are grieving while you're caregiving.
The person is fading in front of you long before they die.
The grief is layered, ongoing, and heavy.

You deserve support.
You cannot do the work of an entire team alone.

Daily Habits That Keep You From Breaking

Eat real food.
Your body needs fuel, not crumbs over the sink.

Drink water.
Hydration affects your patience, cognition, and emotional stability.

Move your body.
Walk. Stretch. Go outside. Five minutes counts.

Breathe on purpose.
Deep breaths pull your nervous system back from the edge.

Ask for help before you collapse.
Don't wait until you're burnt to ash.

Cry when you need to.
Tears release pressure. Let them.

Do one thing a day that belongs to you.
Music. A shower. A show. A snack. A moment of quiet. Something that reminds you that you're alive outside of caregiving.

Scripts That Get You Through Hard Moments

When they're agitated:
"You're safe. I'm right here."

When they repeat questions:
"We're okay. I've got everything handled."

When they refuse care:
"Let's try this together."

When they accuse you of something:

"I'm sorry you're feeling that way. Let me help."

When they think someone is in the house:
"That sounds scary. I'll check and make sure everything is safe."

When they want to "go home":
"We can rest here for a bit first."

When they're scared at night:
"You're not alone. I'm staying close."

When they panic because you're leaving:
"I'll be back soon. You're safe until I return."

Scripts aren't manipulation. Scripts are bridges. You are speaking to the emotional brain, not the logical one.

Getting Support Without Feeling Like You're Failing

Ask people for specific tasks:

- "Can you come sit with her Thursday from one to three?"

- "Can you pick up groceries this week?"

- "Can you handle the pharmacy run?"

General offers never help.
Specific asks do.

Rotate support.
Family, friends, paid caregivers, respite services.

Let go of the idea that you must do everything.
You can't.
And you shouldn't.

Bring in help long before crisis.
Memory care, home health, hospice—these are lifelines, not failures.

Signs You Need Immediate Support

If you see yourself in any of these, it's time to bring in help now:

- You're sleeping less than five hours.

- You're snapping at your person.

- You're crying regularly.

- You're losing weight or overeating.

- You're feeling constantly overwhelmed.

- You're forgetting your own tasks or appointments.

- You're isolating.

- You feel resentment building.

- You can't leave them alone for even a moment.

- You're afraid something bad will happen.

- You're afraid you won't survive this.

These are not weaknesses.
These are indicators that you've been carrying too much for too long.

The Bottom Line

Caregiving is brutal and beautiful.
It is exhausting and sacred.
It is trauma and devotion braided together.

You matter too.
Your needs matter.
Your rest matters.

Your health matters.
Your identity matters.

Nothing about dementia is simple.
But here is the truth every caregiver needs carved into their bones:

You are not meant to survive this alone.

CHAPTER 15
CAREGIVER GUILT VS.
CAREGIVER RESPONSIBILITY

Caregiver guilt is one of the most powerful forces in dementia care — and one of the most misunderstood.

It's the quiet voice that says:
"I should be doing more".
"I shouldn't feel this way".
"Other people handle this better than I do".
"If I were stronger, I wouldn't need help".

Caregiver responsibility, on the other hand, is grounded in reality.

And dementia forces those two things into constant collision.

Let's Name the Difference Clearly

Caregiver guilt is emotional.
It's rooted in love, fear, history, expectations, and the story you tell yourself about what a "good" caregiver should be.

Caregiver responsibility is practical.
It's rooted in safety, capacity, sustainability, and what the disease actually requires — not what you wish it required.

The problem is that guilt is loud, dramatic, and relentless.
Responsibility is quiet, steady, and often ignored.

And dementia thrives when guilt is in charge.

What Guilt Sounds Like

Caregiver guilt says things like:

- "They took care of me — I owe them everything".

- "If I loved them enough, this wouldn't feel so hard".

- "Other people manage without complaining".

- "I promised I'd never put them in a facility".

- "I should be able to handle this".

- "If I stop, something bad will happen".

Guilt doesn't care if you're exhausted.
Guilt doesn't care if you're sick.
Guilt doesn't care if the situation is unsafe.
Guilt only cares about punishment.

And guilt lies.

What Responsibility Actually Is

Caregiver responsibility is not martyrdom.

It does not mean:

- sacrificing your health

- losing your identity

- absorbing endless emotional abuse

- functioning on zero sleep

- ignoring danger signs

- pretending you're fine when you're not

Responsibility means asking one hard question over and over:

"What is safest, most sustainable, and most humane — for both of us?"

Sometimes the answer is staying home.
Sometimes it's bringing in help.
Sometimes it's memory care.
Sometimes it's hospice.
Sometimes it's stepping back before you break.

Responsibility adapts as the disease progresses.
Guilt refuses to evolve.

The Lie That Traps Caregivers

One of the most damaging beliefs caregivers carry is this:

"If I choose myself at any point, I am abandoning them".

That is false.

You are not abandoning someone by:

- sleeping

- eating

- resting

- asking for help

- setting limits

- admitting something is too much

You are acknowledging reality.

And reality is this:
Dementia requires more care than one person can safely give, indefinitely.

That doesn't make you weak.
That makes you honest.

Love Is Not the Same as Capacity

You can love someone deeply and still not be able to meet their needs alone.

Love does not increase your physical strength.
Love does not eliminate exhaustion.
Love does not override neurological decline.
Love does not make you immune to burnout.

Love motivates care.
Capacity determines how that care happens.

Confusing the two is how caregivers disappear.

When Guilt Is Running the Show

If guilt is in charge, you'll notice patterns like:

- pushing yourself past exhaustion

- ignoring your own health

- feeling resentful but ashamed of it

- snapping and then hating yourself for it

- staying in unsafe situations "a little longer"

- avoiding help because it feels like failure

- measuring your worth by how much you suffer

That is not love.
That is survival mode mixed with fear.

Responsibility Requires Permission — And You Have It

Here is the permission caregivers rarely receive:

You are allowed to change the plan.

You are allowed to say:

- "This is more than I can safely do".

- "I need help".

- "We need more support".

- "This isn't working anymore".

Those statements are not betrayals.
They are acts of protection.

For you.
For them.
For the relationship.

The Truth Most Caregivers Learn Too Late

Caregivers don't regret asking for help too early.

They regret waiting too long.

They regret the injuries.
The breakdowns.
The lost years.
The damage to their own bodies and marriages and mental health.

They regret letting guilt make decisions that

responsibility should have made.

Let This Be the Line You Cross

Guilt asks:
How much can I endure?

Responsibility asks:
What keeps everyone safest and most intact?

One drains you.
The other sustains you.

You are not required to destroy yourself to prove
your love.

You are allowed to care with limits.
You are allowed to choose sustainability over
sacrifice.
You are allowed to protect yourself without
apology.

That is not selfish.
That is responsible caregiving.

And it is enough.

CHAPTER 16
WHAT CAREGIVERS WISH
THEY'D KNOWN SOONER

Caregivers don't usually look back and say, "I wish I loved them more."

They say things like:

- "I wish I'd known this would last longer than I thought".

- "I wish I'd known it was okay to ask for help sooner".

- "I wish I'd known how much this would change me".

- "I wish I'd known I wasn't failing — I was adapting".

This chapter exists so you don't have to learn everything the hard way.
So, here we go.

Dementia Is a Marathon Disguised as a Sprint

Most caregivers begin with the belief that this will be a "phase."
A rough season.
Something they just need to push through.

It's not.

Dementia is long.
It stretches.
It evolves.
It demands more over time, not less.

Caregivers wish they'd known early that pace matters.
Burning yourself out in the first few miles doesn't help anyone at the finish line.

You Will Grieve While They're Still Alive — And That's Normal

Caregivers are often blindsided by grief that shows up before death.

Grief when:

- they stop recognizing you

- their personality shifts

- their independence disappears

- conversations stop making sense

- roles reverse

Many caregivers think something is wrong with them for feeling grief early.

Nothing is wrong.
This is anticipatory grief.
And it's real.

You're not dramatic.
You're not negative.
You're responding to loss that keeps unfolding.

Love Will Not Fix This — But It Still Matters

Caregivers wish they'd known that love does not cure dementia.

It doesn't slow it.
It doesn't reverse it.

It doesn't make the hard days disappear.

But love still matters — just differently.

Love becomes:

- safety

- tone

- consistency

- presence

- comfort

- dignity

You are no longer preserving who they were.
You are protecting who they are.

That shift changes everything.

You Cannot Do This Alone — No Matter How Capable You Are

Caregivers often pride themselves on being strong, responsible, capable people.

Dementia doesn't care.

It requires:

- physical stamina

- emotional regulation

- constant supervision

- medical management

- behavioral understanding

- contingency planning

No single person can sustainably provide all of that.

Caregivers wish they'd known sooner that needing help is not weakness — it's basic math.

Guilt Will Show Up — But It Doesn't Get to Decide

Caregivers are shocked by how loud guilt becomes.

Guilt about:

- getting frustrated

- wanting breaks

- considering memory care

- missing their old life

- feeling relief when things quiet down

Guilt feels convincing.
It feels moral.
It feels urgent.

But guilt is not a reliable decision-maker.

Caregivers wish they'd known earlier that guilt can exist without being obeyed.

Some Relationships Will Change — And That's Not Your Fault

Dementia strains families.

Some people step up.
Some disappear.
Some criticize from a distance.
Some rewrite history.

Caregivers wish they'd known not to spend so much energy trying to make everyone understand.

Not everyone will.
And that doesn't invalidate your reality.

Protecting your energy becomes part of the care plan.

You Will Lose Parts of Yourself — And You Can Find Them Again

Caregiving reshapes identity.

You may lose:

- spontaneity

- freedom

- confidence

- patience

- parts of your social world

Caregivers often think this loss is permanent.

It's not.

Some parts pause.
Some parts change.
Some parts come back later — stronger, clearer, more grounded.

You are still in there.

Even if you can't reach yourself right now.

There Is No "Right Way" to Do This

Caregivers waste enormous energy comparing themselves to others.

Someone always seems more patient.
More organized.
More selfless.
More composed.

Caregivers wish they'd known sooner that there is no gold standard for dementia caregiving.

There is only:

- safe enough

- kind enough

- sustainable enough

And that is enough.

The End Will Be Complicated — And So Will Your Feelings

Caregivers are rarely prepared for the emotional

aftermath.

Relief.
Sadness.
Emptiness.
Guilt.
Freedom.
Disorientation.

All at once.

Caregivers wish they'd known earlier that mixed emotions do not cancel each other out.
They coexist.

And they don't mean you loved any less.

You Are Doing Better Than You Think

This is the truth caregivers almost never believe while they're in it.

You notice what you did wrong.
You replay your worst moments.
You forget the thousands of quiet acts of care you perform without applause.

Caregivers wish they'd known how much they

mattered while they were still doing it.

Let this be the moment you hear it:

You are not failing.
You are adapting.
You are learning a job no one trains for.
You are carrying something heavy with imperfect
hands.

And you are doing better than you think.

This chapter doesn't exist to make caregiving easier.

It exists to make it less lonely.

And to remind you — again — of something true:

You were never meant to figure this out alone.

CHAPTER 17
HOW DO I KNOW WHEN IT'S TIME FOR MEMORY CARE?

Most people wait WAY too long.

They wait until:

- someone gets hurt

- a caregiver collapses

- finances crash

- behavior becomes dangerous

- their loved one deteriorates

You don't have to wait for rock bottom.

Here are the real signs it may be time.

Sign #1: They're not safe at home, even with help.

Examples:

- wandering

- leaving the stove on

- forgetting to eat

- not recognizing danger

- getting lost in their own house

- sudden aggression or paranoia

- repeated falls

If the home is becoming a hazard more than a refuge, that's a red flag.

Sign #2: You cannot meet their needs without harming your own health.

If the care they require is:

- physically too demanding

- mentally draining

- emotionally breaking you

- keeping you from sleeping

- destroying your ability to function

…then it's no longer "caregiving."

It becomes self-destruction.

And that helps absolutely no one.

Sign #3: You can't leave them alone for even 10 minutes.

If you're living on constant alert — like parenting a toddler who can open doors, but with a hell of a lot more risk — that's unsustainable.

Hypervigilance is not a long-term care plan.
It's a breaking point.

Sign #4: Care needs exceed what one person (or family) can safely do.

Dementia eventually becomes:

- 24/7 supervision

- medication management

- toileting assistance

- mobility help

- behavioral support

- constant redirection

This requires a team, not a hero.

Sign #5: Their medical needs are becoming complex.

Things like:

- diabetes

- heart conditions

- incontinence

- pressure injury risk

- frequent infections

- mobility decline

Memory care has staff trained for this.
Home caregivers are human beings, not medical machines.

Sign #6: Your loved one's dignity is being unintentionally compromised.

Sometimes staying home:

- increases agitation

- increases confusion

- increases dependence

- increases fear

Structured environments often reduce these things. People can actually thrive after placement — more calm, more routine, more support.

Sign #7: You're doing it out of guilt, not out of capacity.

If the ONLY reason you're keeping them home is something like:

- "They took care of me, so I owe them."

- "People will think I abandoned them."

- "My family will judge me."

- "It feels like failing."

…that's not sustainable, and it's not fair to you or to them.

Love does not mean doing everything alone.
Love means doing what's safe.

"But How Do I NOT Feel Like a Monster For Choosing Memory Care?"

Let's get brutally honest.

You feel guilt because you care.

Monsters don't feel guilt.
Caregivers do.

You are not abandoning them.

You are changing the location of their care — not the quality of your love.

This is not the end of your relationship.

It's the beginning of a safer chapter.

You're not choosing memory care OVER them.

You're choosing memory care FOR them.

You're not replacing yourself.

You're reinforcing yourself with a whole damn team.

You are one person.
Dementia requires many.

CHAPTER 18
HOME CARE VS. MEMORY CARE

HOME CARE — Pros

- familiar environment

- comfort

- personalized attention

- one-on-one care

- sense of independence

HOME CARE — Cons

- exhausting for caregivers

- unsafe as disease progresses

- social isolation

- requires constant supervision

- burnout is almost guaranteed

MEMORY CARE — Pros

- 24/7 trained staff

- structured routine

- social stimulation

- medication management

- safe, wander-resistant environment

- professional behavioral support

MEMORY CARE — Cons

- emotional transition

- cost

- family guilt

- adjusting to new surroundings

- occasional resistance from the loved one

How to Choose a GOOD Memory Care Facility

Here are the non-negotiables:

✓ Staff ratio
The lower, the better.
Overworked staff = stressed residents.

✓ Clean, cheerful environment
You should feel peace when you walk in — not
dread.

✓ Communication
Staff should update you, welcome you, and include
you.

✓ Activities that are real
Not a room full of silent people staring at a TV.

✓ Locked, safe, wander-resistant design
Memory care must be built for dementia — not just
"old people."

✓ Consistent staff
Rotating strangers increase confusion.

✓ A director who gives a damn
If leadership sucks, everything sucks.

The Transition:
How to Move Someone to Memory Care Without Breaking Them (or Yourself)

Rule #1: Keep explanations simple.
Too much info = anxiety.

Rule #2: Don't tell them weeks ahead.
They'll forget — and panic daily.

Rule #3: Move in the morning.
Brains are calmer.

Rule #4: Stick around but not too long.
Long goodbyes increase agitation.

Rule #5: Expect an adjustment period.
2–6 weeks is normal.

Rule #6: You are allowed to cry.
It means you're human.

CHAPTER 19
THE DEMENTIA CAREGIVER TOOLKIT

Real Tools for the Days That Break You

This chapter is not here to inspire you.
It's here to help you survive.

Because when dementia is loud, unpredictable, and relentless, what caregivers need most is not platitudes — it's practical tools that actually work in the moment.

This is the toolkit I wish every caregiver had on day one.

GENERAL SAFETY REALITIES CAREGIVERS MUST ACCEPT

If you're wondering, "Is this safe?"
It probably isn't.

Assume they are one step away from danger, even on good days.

Key areas:

- Falls

- Wandering

- Medications

- Cooking

- Bathrooms

Tools:

- Remove throw rugs

- Install grab bars

- Lock or alarm doors

- Simplify the environment

- Supervise medications

Safety is not about control.
It's about prevention.
That's not cruelty.
That's love.

COMMUNICATION TOOLS THAT ACTUALLY WORK

Speak Less.
Mean More.

Dementia processing speed is slower.
Too many words overwhelm the brain.

Use:

- Short sentences

- Simple language

- One idea at a time

Instead of:
"Okay, let's get dressed and then we'll eat and then we need to take your medicine."

Try:
"Let's put on your shirt."
Pause.
"Good. Now your pants."

Clarity lowers anxiety.

Tone Is the Message

Long before words disappear, tone remains.

Speak like you are calm.
Speak like you are confident.
Speak like you are safe.

Even when you're exhausted.
Even when you're scared.

The emotional brain listens when logic can't.

What NOT to Say — Even Though It's Tempting:

- "That didn't happen."

- "You already asked me that."

- "I just told you."

- "You're wrong."

- "Calm down."

These phrases escalate fear, not clarity.

Handling Repetition Without Losing Your Mind

Repetition is not a memory problem.
It's an anxiety problem.

They repeat because:

- They feel unsafe

- They're unsure

- Their brain can't hold reassurance.

Tools That Help:

- Answer calmly, every time

- Write the answer down and point to it

- Use consistent phrases ("You're safe. I've got this.")

- Redirect attention after reassurance

You're not reinforcing the behavior — you're soothing fear.

Validation Before Redirection

Never correct first.
Correcting creates fear.

Validate the feeling, then redirect.

Examples:

- "That sounds frustrating."

- "I can see why you'd feel worried."

- "That makes sense."

Then gently guide:

- "Let's sit over here."

- "Let me help with that."

You're calming the nervous system — not winning an argument.

And arguing with dementia is like yelling at a broken GPS.

When Behavior Escalates

Understand this first, and foremost:

Behavior is communication.

Agitation = fear
Repetition = insecurity
Anger = loss of control
Accusations = confusion
Wandering = searching

Ask yourself:
"What is the unmet need?"

Hunger?
Pain?
Fatigue?
Overstimulation?
Fear?

Fix the cause — not the behavior.

Calming Tools in the Moment

- Lower your voice

- Slow your movements

- Stand to the side, not face-to-face

- Give space, not commands

- Offer a familiar object

- Use rhythm (rocking, humming, gentle repetition)

Do NOT match their energy.
Absorb it.

Managing Agitation, Sundowning & Big Emotions

Agitation usually means overstimulation or unmet needs.

Common triggers:

- Fatigue

- Hunger

- Pain

- Noise

- Too many choices

- Changes in routine

What Helps:

- Dim lights in the evening

- Reduce noise

- Keep routines predictable

- Offer comfort objects

- Use music they recognize

- Sit beside them instead of standing over them

When emotions rise, logic is already gone.
Your job is to lower the temperature, not explain the weather.

Delusions, Hallucinations & False Beliefs

Again, this is one of the hardest parts.

They may believe:

- Someone is stealing

- Someone is in the house

- They're not home

- They're late for work

- A spouse is alive or unfaithful

The Rule:
Do not argue with their reality.

Try:

- "That sounds upsetting."

- "I'll check on that."

- "You're safe right now."

Correcting dementia often feels cruel — because to their brain, it is.

Bathing, Dressing & Personal Care Without a Battle

Personal care feels threatening when the brain can't sequence steps.

Tips:

- Warm the room

- Explain each step slowly

- Use towels for modesty

- Offer choices only when they're simple

- Stop if agitation rises

If today doesn't work, try again later. Care doesn't have to happen on your schedule to count.

SAFE FEEDING & SWALLOWING BASICS

Why Mealtimes Change — and What Actually Helps

Swallowing is a neurological process.
When dementia progresses, the brain slowly loses the ability to coordinate the muscles needed to chew, move food, and protect the airway.

This is not laziness.
This is not refusal.
This is not someone being dramatic.

It is the brain forgetting how to eat.

Early Warning Signs of Swallowing Difficulty

Pay attention to these signs — they matter:

- Coughing or throat clearing during or after meals

- Pocketing food in the cheeks

- Wet, gurgly, or hoarse voice after swallowing

- Long or exhausting mealtimes

- Frequent pneumonia or chest infections

- Unexplained weight loss

- Watery eyes while eating

- Food remaining in the mouth after swallowing

These are not "quirks."
They are safety signals.

If you notice them, adjustments should happen immediately.

Safer Feeding Strategies

Position matters.
Always sit them upright — feet supported, head

midline. Before, during, and after meals.

Pacing matters.
Slow is safer.
Small bites.
Wait for the swallow before offering the next.

Food choice matters.

Safer options include:

- Soft foods

- Moist foods

- Warm foods (often easier to sense)

Riskier foods include:

- Dry or crumbly foods

- Mixed textures (cereal with milk, soup with chunks)

- Tough meats

- Super sticky foods that don't break down easily

Liquids should only be thickened if recommended

by an SLP.

Thicker is NOT always safer. For the love of God, read that again.

Feeding With Dignity

Never feed over someone.
Sit with them.
Eat together when possible.

Offer reassurance.
Speak softly.
Wipe gently.
Maintain eye contact.

If they push food away:
Stop.
Pause.
Try again later.

Forcing food increases fear and aspiration risk.

When Eating Begins to Fade

As dementia advances, appetite naturally decreases.
The body no longer processes hunger the same way.

At this stage:

- Nutrition becomes secondary to comfort

- Favorite tastes matter more than calories

- Finger foods are golden

- Small sips, ice chips, and comfort foods are appropriate

- Mealtime becomes about connection, not completion

This is not starvation.
This is the body following the disease process.

The Hard Truth Caregivers Need

Aspiration risk increases as dementia progresses.
Weight loss is common.
Feeding will change.

Your job is not to "make them eat."
Your job is to keep them safe, comfortable, and respected.

Love does not mean pushing past the body's limits.
Love means honoring what the body can still do.

And sometimes, that means letting go of what

eating used to look like.

THE DAILY ROUTINE TEMPLATE

Consistency Prevents Meltdowns

MORNING

- Bathroom / hygiene

- Simple breakfast

- Light activity (stretching, walking, sorting)

MIDDAY

- Lunch

- Rest time (non-negotiable)

- Calm activity (music, folding towels, photo albums)

EVENING

- Early dinner

- Low stimulation time

- Bedtime routine (same order *every* night)

THE RULE:

Predictability gives the brain something to hold onto.

THE CAREGIVER SELF-PRESERVATION KIT

You are not optional.

Burnout signs:

- Irritability

- Emotional numbness

- Poor sleep

- Resentment

- Crying easily

- Brain fog

- Feeling trapped

If you see three or more — you need help now.

Not later.
Not "after this phase."

Now.

Read this slowly.
You will:

- Lose your patience

- Say the wrong thing

- Cry in private

- Wish this wasn't your life

None of that makes you a bad caregiver.

It makes you human.

Dementia is not a test you pass or fail.
It is something you survive.

Boundaries You Are Allowed to Set

"I can't do this alone."
"I need help."
"I need rest."
"I can't be available 24/7."
"I need support."

These are not selfish statements.

They are survival statements.

The Truth At The Core of this Toolkit

You were never meant to figure this out by instinct.
The disease is too complex.
The demands are too heavy.
The cost is too high.

Tools don't make you cold.
They make you steady.

And steadiness is what dementia care requires.

You are not failing.
You are adapting.
And that is strength.

FROM THE FIELD: CLARICE: THE SECRETARY WORKPLACE DELUSION

There was a gentleman I worked with for years — blunt, charismatic without trying, sharp in flashes, and fully committed to whatever reality his brain decided to clock into that day. I adored him.

One afternoon, while I was finishing a session with another patient, I heard a wheelchair rolling up behind me with purpose. He stopped right at my shoulder, cleared his throat like a man about to deliver a TED Talk, and said:

"Clarice, when you finish whatever it is you're doing, I need you to come to my office so we can discuss some things."

Clarice.
A name I have never had. Not even close.

But he said it with such authority — such CEO energy — that I simply nodded like I'd been Clarice every day of my adult life.

I wrapped up my session and followed him down

the hallway… not to an office, but to his room. He maneuvered into place like a boss rolling back into headquarters. I sat down across from him and asked gently:

"Alright, what's going on?"

That's when I received a full-blown performance evaluation.

He told me he didn't understand why I was struggling with the tasks he'd assigned me. He said he'd given me very clear instructions. He said if he needed to replace me, he absolutely would. He was disappointed — truly disappointed — in my work as his secretary.

So I did what dementia care requires every single day:
I stepped fully into his world.

I apologized for my "poor performance."
I promised to do better.
I asked him to show me exactly what he expected.

I grabbed papers from his bedside table and pretended to file them.

I took "notes" on imaginary tasks.

I reorganized a stack of magazines like they were confidential files.

I nodded seriously as he outlined my job duties.

And as I leaned into his world, something softened.

His frustration melted into relief.

His tone eased.

He reclaimed control — authority — identity.

All the things dementia had been stripping from him, piece by piece.

By the end of our "meeting," he thanked me for listening.

He apologized for being harsh, but reminded me — with great dignity — that he was the boss.

A few days later, when his daughter visited, I casually asked about his work history. I wanted to understand the world he'd taken me into. I asked if there had ever been a secretary. A coworker named Clarice. A job that required one.

She laughed.

No secretary.

No Clarice.
Not then, not ever.

The entire storyline — the office, the authority, the job title, the frustration, the need to "correct my work" — all of it came from the world his brain built for him that day.

But here's the beautiful thing:

The delusion wasn't really about me being Clarice.
It was about him needing to feel capable again.
Competent again.
Important again.
HIMSELF again.

And I got to meet him there.

Dementia reshapes reality, yes.
But sometimes it creates these small, sacred universes where connection still lives, humor still breathes, and humanity still finds you — even when memory doesn't.

Clarice wasn't real.
The bond was.

PART 4
THE END OF THE ROAD

No one wants to arrive at this part of the journey.
Most people hope they'll never need these pages —
and yet, almost everyone does.

This section exists because the end of dementia is
often more frightening in imagination than it is in
reality.
Families are rarely told what to expect, what is
normal, or how much of what they're feeling is
human — not failure.

This part of the book is not about giving up.
It's about understanding what comes next.
It's about comfort, dignity, honesty, and love when
the disease has taken all it can.

You don't have to read this section all at once.
You don't have to read it until you're ready.

But when the time comes, this is meant to be a light
in a place that often feels unbearably dark.

CHAPTER 20
END OF LIFE & HOSPICE

No one wants to talk about the end.

Not families.

Not friends.

Not even most professionals.

But you deserve the truth before you get blindsided by it.

You deserve to understand what's coming so you're not walking into the darkest part of this journey without a light.

Hospice is not giving up.

Death is not failure.

The end is not abandonment.

This is what dementia looks like when the final chapter begins to turn.

What Dying from Dementia Actually Looks Like

People do not die because "the dementia got too bad."

They die because the brain can no longer run the

body.

In the final phase, the brain forgets how to swallow, how to sense hunger, how to regulate breathing, how to stay awake, how to fight infections, how to keep the body going.
The body begins shutting down.
Slowly.
Quietly.
Naturally.

This is not suffering.
This is biology.

Signs That the End Is Approaching

These changes unfold over weeks to months.

- Increasing sleep

- Eating less or refusing food

- Noticeable weight loss

- Difficulty swallowing

- Minimal speech

- Irregular breathing

- Cool hands and feet

- Detaching from the environment

It is not giving up.
It is the body transitioning.

What Hospice Really Is

Hospice is comfort.
Hospice is dignity.
Hospice is symptom management.
Hospice is emotional support.
Hospice is a team.
Hospice is peace.

It is not killing someone.
It is not forcing death.
It is not abandoning care.

Hospice is love in its final form.

What You Will Feel in This Stage

You will feel heartbreak.
You will feel tenderness.
You will feel dread.
You will feel relief.

You will feel guilt for the relief.
You will feel exhausted.
You will feel overwhelmed.
You will feel love so fierce it nearly breaks you.

Nothing about your emotional response is wrong.
Nothing.

What You Should Do in the Final Days

Talk to them.
Touch them gently.
Play familiar music.
Keep the room calm.
Let hospice manage symptoms.
Let yourself feel what you feel.

Hearing is the last sense to go.
Your voice is comfort.

What It's Like When They Take Their Last Breath

It is usually quiet.
It is usually gentle.
It is usually peaceful.

A long exhale.
A loosened expression.
A stillness that settles into the room.

Not dramatic.
Not violent.
Just a body finishing its final task.

What Happens to You Afterwards

This is the moment caregivers fall apart.
This is the moment your body collapses after
months or years of holding tension.
This is when grief becomes real.

You may feel emptiness.
You may feel shock.
You may feel freedom.
You may feel guilt for that freedom.
You may feel deep, aching love.
You may feel lost.

Your nervous system doesn't know the crisis is
over.
It will take time.

The Truth You Need Most

You did not fail.
You did not choose wrong.
You did not give up.

Dementia ends with death.
That is the disease.
Not your doing.

You walked them all the way to the end with love.
That matters.
More than anything.

CHAPTER 21
GRIEF AFTER DEMENTIA

Grief in dementia does not start at the funeral.
It starts with the first forgotten story, the first
confused look, the first moment you realize
something is wrong.
You lose them slowly and then suddenly.

This grief is layered.
This grief is relentless.
This grief is strange.
This grief is lonely.

And after they die, the grief doesn't stop.
It simply changes shape.

The First Grief

The grief of noticing.
The grief of knowing something is slipping.
The grief before you know the name of the enemy.

You don't call it grief then, but it is.
It is the beginning.

The Slow-Motion Grief

Losing someone in fragments is unlike any loss on earth.
Every stage of decline is another tiny funeral.
Every shift is another goodbye.

You lose their stories.
Their independence.
Their confidence.
Their personality.
Their routines.
Their abilities.

You grieve while they're still alive.
You learn to smile through sorrow.

The Caregiver-Shaped Grief

You lose yourself, too.

Your freedom.
Your patience.
Your health.
Your identity.
Your social life.
Your energy.

And then you grieve the version of you that existed before dementia reshaped you.

Pre-Death Grief

You know the end is coming.
You feel it.
You dread it.
And you also crave relief from the suffering—for them and for you.
That mix of emotions is normal, human, and brutally honest.

After-Death Grief

This is the one no one warns you about.

Your body keeps waiting for the next crisis.
You wake up bracing for something that isn't coming.
You no longer know who you are without caregiving.

You feel untethered.
You feel empty.
You feel free and guilty for feeling free.
You feel broken open.

And you rebuild slowly.

In layers.

In waves.

Guilt Grief

Caregivers carry guilt like a second skin.

Not patient enough.

Not strong enough.

Not present enough.

Not fast enough.

Not loving enough.

But here is the truth:

You did the best you could in a situation no one is equipped for.

Your love stayed.

Your presence mattered.

That is enough.

The Love That Remains

The love does not die.

The love becomes memory.

The love becomes story.

The love becomes the part of you that survived all

of this.

You didn't just lose them.
You gained a deeper, harder, more sacred
understanding of love itself.

FROM THE FIELD: THE MAN WHO DIDN'T LIKE DOGS... UNTIL HE LOVED ONE

There was a gentleman I worked with for a few years — one of those men who seemed made of equal parts blunt honesty, stubborn charm, and a lifetime of grit. Before I tell you this story, you need to know one thing: I worked side-by-side with my best friend, Theodore.

Theodore was a 200-pound French Mastiff — a walking emotional-support sofa with jowls. Most of my patients adored him and preferred him to me. At least once a day I'd hear:

"Where's Theodore? We don't need you — we want HIM."

Honestly? Fair.

But this man?
He took one look at Theodore on the first day and said:

"I don't like dogs. I don't like dog hair. I don't care to see him."

Clear. Direct. Brutal.
So, I respected it and kept Theodore out of his line of sight.

But something shifted — slowly at first, then all at once.

One afternoon I heard a wheelchair rolling fast behind me. It was him. No hello. No small talk. Just urgency — like the FBI had issued a canine alert:

"Hey. Is Theodore here? I thought I just saw him go that way."

Sir... what?

The man who hated dogs had flipped the script so hard he practically threw the whole book.

Soon, he was rolling around the building every day like Theodore's personal security detail, asking everyone, "Y'all seen that dog?"
If I came to work without Theodore, he was offended:

"Well, if I'd known you weren't bringing the good one, I wouldn't have gotten out of bed."

Eventually he became Theodore's unofficial photographer, hype man, and snack dealer. I'd catch him slipping crackers or dinner rolls under the table like contraband. Sometimes I'd find icing or crumbs crusted in Theodore's facial folds and think, What fresh hell is this?

One day a nurse casually said,
"Oh yeah, he fed Theodore all the treats he made this week."

THE TREATS HE MADE.

Excuse me?

Turns out he had been requesting ingredients from family members so he could handcraft "dog biscuits" in his room. Not real biscuits — I'm talking:
saltines smothered in peanut butter
mashed cake
mystery blends of God-knows-what

And he fed them to Theodore proudly, behind my

back, like he was running a black-market bakery.

Meanwhile, I'm over here taking Theodore to the vet, doing the concerned-dog-mom routine, getting side-eyes about his weight, putting him on prescription food, swearing I'm following the diet to the letter…

Turns out I was being sabotaged by a man in a wheelchair with peanut butter and a dream.

Then came the moment that knocked the air out of my chest.

He was sitting on the porch with his daughter, who had a grocery bag on her lap. I joked, "Ooh, did you bring him some goodies?"

Before she could answer, he announced, "Yep, she brought me stuff."

She gave me a look like, Sorry, he's being rude, then said softly:

"He's never liked peanut butter, but he keeps asking me to bring him some … so I do."

And that's when it hit me.

He wasn't asking for peanut butter for himself.
He was asking for ingredients…
for Theodore.

My throat tightened.
This man — who had sworn he didn't like dogs —
had been crafting love in the form of peanut-butter-
covered saltines.

And the final blow?

One day he handed me his phone for help, and on
the screen was a Google search typed slowly,
imperfectly, heartbreakingly:

"how too make dog treets at home is peanut buttr
good for dogs"

I had to look away for a second.

Because this man wasn't just giving my dog scraps.
He was trying to learn what was safe.
He wanted to take care of him — intentionally,
gently, fiercely.

He never said, "I love that dog."
He never admitted he'd changed his mind.
But he didn't need to.

It was in the stolen cake.
The peanut butter.
The homemade "biscuits."
The photos.
The Google searches typed with trembling fingers.

He adored Theodore.
And Theodore adored him right back.

This work gives you relationships you never see coming.
It teaches you that connection finds a way — even through dementia, even through grumpiness, even through stubbornness so thick you could slice it.

Some of the most unexpected bonds I've ever witnessed began with someone saying,
"I don't like dogs."

And ended with them loving one more purely than they ever expected.

PART 5
TALKING TO KIDS & FAMILY DYNAMICS

Dementia doesn't just affect one person.
It ripples outward — through families, through relationships, through generations.

Kids sense it before they understand it.
Families feel it before they name it.
Old dynamics resurface.
New tensions form.
Roles shift in ways no one trained for.

This section is about navigating those ripple effects with honesty, clarity, and compassion — for children who need truth they can hold, and for families trying to survive something that exposes every crack.

There is no perfect script.
But there are better ways to talk, listen, and protect one another through the chaos.

CHAPTER 22
EXPLAINING THE UNEXPLAINABLE TO CHILDREN

This can be bite-sized hell.
Talking to kids about dementia and death is one of the moments caregivers fear most — not because children are fragile, but because adults are.

We're afraid of saying the wrong thing.
We're afraid of breaking something in them.
We're afraid of answering questions we don't yet have answers for ourselves.

Here's the truth most people don't tell you:

Children don't need perfect explanations.
They need honest ones.
They need calm adults.
They need safety, repetition, and permission to feel.

This part of the journey isn't about finding the "right words."
It's about giving kids enough truth so silence doesn't do more harm than honesty.

If you feel clumsy, emotional, unsure, or scared going into these conversations — that doesn't mean you're doing it wrong.

It means you care.
Kids feel everything.
They notice the tension in the room, the whispered conversations, the way adults are suddenly softer, sadder, distracted.
What they don't have is the language to make sense of it.

Your job isn't to protect kids from the truth.
Your job is to give them the truth in a way their brain and heart can process.

Bottom line:
Kids don't need perfection.
They need honesty, clarity, and safety.

If you need a little framework, here are some basic examples you can follow for each developmental stage:

Ages 3–6

"Their brain is sick. The part that helps them

remember and understand things isn't working well. They still love you, and they are safe."

Simple. Gentle. True.

Ages 7–10

"Dementia makes the brain stop working the way it used to. That's why they get confused or say things that don't make sense. They are not doing it on purpose. Their brain is changing."

Clear and comforting.

Ages 11–14

"You're going to see changes. Dementia affects memory, thinking, emotions, and sometimes behavior. It's normal to feel sad, confused, or frustrated."

Honest without being overwhelming.

Ages 15–18

"The disease is progressing. You'll see more confusion, more need for help, and eventually physical changes. None of this is their fault or your responsibility. Whatever you feel is okay."

Respectful. Real.

How To Help All Kids Feel Safe, Regardless of Age

- Establish predictable routines.

- Let them express big feelings without correction.

- Don't force hugs or interactions.

- Explain behaviors in real time:

- "She's not mad at you; she's confused."

- Encourage connection through activities, not conversations.
  (Drawing, music, sitting together.)

Kids don't need the adult version of dementia. They need the child-sized one.

What Not To Say – Even When You Mean Well

Some phrases are commonly used to "protect" children — but they often create confusion, fear, or guilt instead.

Try to avoid:

- "They're just sleeping."
  (Sleep can suddenly become scary.)

- "God needed them."
  (Can create anger, fear, or confusion about faith.)

- "Everything happens for a reason."
  (Invalidates pain.)

- "Be strong."
  (Teaches emotional suppression.)

- "Don't cry."
  (Teaches that grief is wrong.)

Kids don't need protection from truth.
They need protection from confusion.

Clear, calm language builds safety — even when the truth is hard.

When Kids Ask The Same Question Again (And Again)

They will.

Tomorrow.
Next week.
Six months from now.

Answer it again.
With the same calm voice.
With the same simple words.

Repetition is how children process grief — just like repetition is how adults with dementia process the world.

It's not manipulation.
It's not attention-seeking.
It's integration.

Each time they ask, their brain is trying to make sense of something that feels too big to hold all at once.
Your steady response becomes their anchor.

WHAT I WISH PEOPLE KNEW FROM THE BEGINNING – IN A NUTSHELL

Dementia doesn't stay contained inside one person. It expands astronomically outward — through children, siblings, spouses, in-laws, old wounds, unspoken expectations, and family roles that were set decades before the diagnosis ever existed.

How a family communicates, avoids, controls, supports, or collapses under stress suddenly matters more than ever.

The disease doesn't create dysfunction — it exposes it.

And understanding those dynamics isn't about blame.

It's about surviving this with as much clarity, compassion, and self-protection as possible.

CHAPTER 23
THE MESSY REALITY OF
FAMILY DYNAMICS

If you want to see a family's true personality, put one of them in a dementia journey.

People don't become different during caregiving.
They become *more* of who they already were.

The overfunctioner overfunctions.
The avoider disappears.
The martyr suffers loudly.
The peacemaker tries to keep the peace in a war zone.
The angry one gets angrier.
The "I live far away" sibling suddenly has opinions about everything.
The financially irresponsible sibling steals meds or money.
The perfectionist wants daily charts and updates.
Everyone regresses into childhood roles.

This is normal.
Not fun.
Not fair.

But normal.

Why Dementia Turns Families Against Each Other

Dementia doesn't create family dysfunction.
It exposes it under pressure.

Fear, anticipatory grief, exhaustion, guilt, denial, and old family roles all collide at once — often without warning.

People respond based on how they cope with stress, not how much they love.

Some avoid.
Some control.
Some criticize.
Some disappear.
Some overfunction.

This doesn't excuse harm — but it explains why things get messy so fast.

Understanding this won't fix everything.
But it may help you stop taking family behavior personally when you're already carrying too much.

What You Cannot Do:

- You cannot make everyone contribute.

- You cannot make siblings apologize or grow up.

- You cannot force shared burden.

- You cannot fix old wounds in the middle of a crisis.

- You cannot be the entire care team alone.

What You Can Do:

- Set boundaries.

- Delegate specific tasks.

- Document everything.

- Communicate clearly and consistently.

- Protect your own mental health.

- Ask for outside support early.

Common Family Conflicts – And How to Handle Them

Conflict #1: "You're doing too much."
Answer: "I'm doing what's necessary. Help me or don't — but please don't undermine me."

Conflict #2: "You're not doing enough."
Answer: "Come spend a full day with me and let's reassess."

Conflict #3: "I don't believe they're that bad."
Answer: "Visit more. Observe more. Trust what I'm telling you."

Conflict #4: "Why wasn't I consulted?"
Answer: "Because decisions must be made quickly. You're included now."

Conflict #5: The will/estate/future-fears spiral
Answer: "Let's set up a meeting with a professional so this isn't emotional warfare."

The Most Important Lesson

You cannot control your family.
You can only control how you navigate them.

You are not responsible for managing everyone else's emotions.

Your job is not to keep the peace at the cost of your sanity.
Your job is not to absorb everyone's fear, denial, or guilt.

Your job is to protect the person living with dementia — and yourself.

Some conversations will land softly.
Some won't.
Some family members will step up.
Some won't.

That doesn't mean you failed.
It means dementia touched more than one life at a time.

You're allowed to set boundaries.
You're allowed to choose safety over approval.
You're allowed to step back from chaos.

Love doesn't require self-destruction.

FROM THE FIELD: THE WOMAN WHO HUMBLED ME AND MY WRINKLES

There was a woman I worked with who carried about six different personalities inside one body — all of them blunt, hilarious, stubborn, and somehow still lovable. She could argue with a wall and win. She had opinions about everything, even things no one asked her about. And depending on the day, she was either fully present or living in an entirely different universe.

One afternoon, she looked at me carefully — studying my face like she was choosing a horse at the Kentucky Derby — and before I could even say hello, she said:

"Well, I mean, I know you're older than I am, but I was only wondering because… you look like you could use some makeup in certain spots of your face. You really could use some. I don't know if anyone taught you that back in your day."

Ma'am…

She was 50 years older than me.
FIFTY.

I just stood there blinking like a confused cartoon character while she looked at me like she was doing me a favor.

So naturally, I swallowed what was left of my pride and said:

"Well… would you like to teach me? Because clearly I need some help."

She nodded — very seriously — as if she'd been waiting her whole life to be asked. She gave me "pointers," which were mostly critiques, but honestly? I deserved them. I just didn't know I deserved them until she told me.

Another day, I found her sitting by the front walkway, staring into the distance like she was waiting for a bus that hadn't existed since 1974. I sat next to her and asked how her day was going.

"Oh, it was great," she said. "I just finished my part in the church and now I'm waiting for my parents to pick me up."

Her parents had been gone for decades.

But I didn't correct her.
I didn't pull her back into our world.
I stepped into hers.

"Okay," I said quietly. "I'll wait with you."

Some days she could tell me every detail about her children — their jobs, their families — and she'd be exactly right. Other days, she'd mix everyone up like a deck of cards. Some days she didn't want to look in a mirror because she didn't want to know if she "looked old." Some days she argued just to argue. Some days she was lost. And some days she was crystal clear.

She was a handful.
And I adored her.

Because underneath all the stubbornness and sass and accidental insults, she trusted me. She let me sit in her worlds with her — whichever one she happened to be in that day.

And she humbled me in the best way possible.

PART 6
WHAT COMES AFTER

Dementia doesn't end neatly.

Whether the journey ends with death, placement, or a slow loosening of the role you carried for so long, there is always an after — and it's rarely discussed.

This part of the book is about what happens when the crisis quiets, the vigilance softens, and you're left standing in a life that no longer looks the way it did before dementia took over.

It's about grief, yes — but also identity, rebuilding, and learning how to live in a body and a mind that have been shaped by caregiving.

There is no right timeline.
No correct way to heal.
No checklist for becoming yourself again.

There is only the next chapter — and the permission to step into it.

I'll Put This Bluntly:
This Is When The Caregiving Stops – But You Don't

They (KIND OF) prepare you for diagnosis.
For caregiving.

For decline.
For crisis.
For loss.

But almost no one talks about what happens after.

After the appointments stop.
After the constant state of readiness ends.
After the phone stops ringing.
After the routines disappear
After the role that defined your days — and nights
— is suddenly gone.

Whether your person has died, moved into full-time
care, or reached a place where your role has
fundamentally changed, there comes a moment
when the storm quiets.

And that quiet can be terrifying.

This part of the journey doesn't come with
instructions.
There is no checklist.
No timeline.
No "right" way to move forward.
Some people expect relief and are startled by grief.
Others expect grief and are confused by numbness,

restlessness, or even moments of peace.

All of it is normal.

You didn't just care for someone with dementia.
You reorganized your life around it.
Your nervous system adapted to constant alert.
Your identity shifted.
Your relationships changed.
Your sense of time, safety, and self were reshaped.

So when the caregiving chapter ends, you don't simply "go back to normal."

There is no normal to go back to.

There is only what comes next.

This section is not about "moving on."
It's about learning how to live again without erasing what mattered.

It's about understanding why your body still feels on edge even when the crisis has passed.
Why quiet feels loud.
Why rest feels unfamiliar.
Why joy can feel disloyal.
Why guilt shows up when you least expect it.

It's about rebuilding a life that makes room for both grief and relief.

For memory and meaning.

For who you were before — and who you are now.

You don't have to rush this part.

You don't have to get it "right."

And you don't have to do it alone.

This is the chapter after survival.

The chapter after holding everything together.

The chapter where you learn how to stand without constant weight on your shoulders.

This is not the end of your story.

It's the beginning of a different one.

CHAPTER 24
REBUILDING LIFE AFTER DEMENTIA

Rebuilding life after dementia is not about "moving on."

It's about learning how to exist in a body and mind that spent a long time in survival mode.

For months or years, your nervous system was calibrated for crisis.
You were listening for falls, wandering, phone calls, breathing changes, emergencies, agitation, fear.
You learned how to live with one ear always open and one eye always watching.

And now… that vigilance has nowhere to go.

So if you feel unsettled, restless, exhausted, numb, guilty, or strangely disconnected from the quiet — that is not weakness.

That is your nervous system slowly realizing the emergency is over.

The Aftermath No One Warns You About

After dementia caregiving ends — whether through death, placement, or role transition — many caregivers expect relief to arrive neatly.

Instead, what shows up can look like:

- emotional whiplash

- grief mixed with relief

- guilt for feeling lighter

- exhaustion that hits after the adrenaline fades

- anxiety with no obvious trigger

- a loss of identity

- difficulty relaxing

- trouble making decisions

- feeling untethered

- wondering, "Who am I now?"

None of this means you did something wrong.

It means your body hasn't caught up to reality yet.

You lived in a constant state of "what if."
It takes time to learn "what now."

You Are Not Broken — You Are Decompressing

Caregivers don't fall apart because they're weak.

They fall apart because they finally can.

When the crisis ends, the body releases what it's been holding. That release can feel like grief, anger, sadness, emptiness, or even panic.
Sometimes all at once.

This is not regression.
This is decompression.

Healing often looks messier than survival.

Letting Go of the Role – Without Letting Go of the Love

Caregiving becomes an identity.

You weren't just helping someone — you were responsible for them.

Their safety.
Their comfort.
Their dignity.
Their survival.

When that responsibility ends, it can feel like:

- abandonment

- disloyalty

- loss of purpose

- guilt for resting

- guilt for laughing

- guilt for planning a future

But here's the truth:

You did not abandon them.
You completed something sacred.

Your love does not disappear just because your role changed.

Love doesn't require constant suffering to remain valid.

Rebuilding Happens Slowly — On Purpose

Rebuilding life after dementia is not about big changes right away.

It's about small permissions.

Permission to rest without justification.
Permission to say no without explanation.
Permission to enjoy something without apology.
Permission to not know what's next yet.

You don't need a five-year plan.
You need breathing room.

Start With These Gentle Foundations

1. Regulate your body before fixing your life.
   Sleep.
   Hydration.
   Gentle movement.
   Regular meals.
   Quiet moments.
   Your nervous system needs consistency before it can handle decisions.

2. Expect delayed grief.
   Grief may show up weeks or months later
   — sometimes triggered by ordinary
   moments.
   This is normal.

3. Separate guilt from responsibility.
   You may feel guilty even when you did
   everything right.
   Guilt does not mean you failed.

4. Rebuild identity in pieces.
   You don't have to "find yourself."
   You get to reintroduce yourself to yourself
   — slowly.

5. Allow joy without permission slips.
Joy does not erase love.
Peace does not negate grief.
Relief does not make you cruel.

You Don't Have to Honor Them by Staying Broken

Some caregivers feel pressure to remain exhausted
or sad — as if healing somehow dishonors the
person they loved.

It doesn't.

You honored them by showing up.
You honored them by staying.
You honored them by loving them through the hardest version of the disease.

You don't need to bleed forever to prove that.

This Is Not the End — It's Integration

Rebuilding life after dementia is not about forgetting.

It's about integrating:

- who you were before

- who you became during caregiving

- who you are allowed to be now

All of those versions belong.

You survived something that changes people.
It would be extremely strange if you emerged unchanged.

But you are still here.

Still capable.
Still worthy of rest, meaning, and connection.

You don't have to rush forward.
You don't have to go backward.
You are allowed to stand exactly where you are —
and take the next step when your body is ready.

This is not weakness.

This is recovery.

FINAL PART
THE LETTERS

These letters are placed here—together,
uninterrupted—because they speak to two VERY
different places a caregiver can be standing:
in the storm, or in the aftermath.

They are meant to be read whenever you need
them.
They are meant to hit where you're hurting.
They are meant to sit with you when no one else
knows how.

LETTER TO THE CAREGIVER STILL IN THE STORM

You're in it right now.

The long nights.
The confusion.
The arguing.
The repetition.
The fear.
The responsibility that feels heavier than anything one person should have to hold.

You are living inside a season that no one prepared you for.
A season without rest, without certainty, without a clear end date.
A season where you wake up every morning already exhausted.
I want you to hear me:

You are not weak.
You are not failing.
You are not supposed to "handle this better."
You are a human being carrying an inhuman load.

You are doing the job of ten people.
You are loving someone through a disease designed to dismantle everything familiar.
You are stepping into every moment as the anchor, the interpreter, the protector, the compass, the soft landing.

You keep going even when you're overstimulated, overtired, overextended, and overwhelmed.

You're in the storm — and you're still here.

That matters.
That counts.
That is strength.
That is love.
That is devotion in its rawest form.

You don't have to be perfect.
You don't have to know what you're doing.
You don't have to smile through it.
You don't have to pretend you're fine.

You only have to keep showing up the way you already are:
messy, tired, angry, gentle, scared, hopeful, and human.

That is more than enough.

You are more than enough.

And even if the world never fully understands what you carry, I do.

I see your courage.
I see your exhaustion.
I see the way you love someone who doesn't always recognize you.
I see the way you fight for someone who cannot fight for themselves.

You are doing the extraordinary inside an impossible situation.

Keep breathing.
Keep standing.
Keep taking it one moment at a time.

The storm won't last forever —
but until it passes, I'm right here with you.

LETTER TO THE CAREGIVER WHO JUST LOST SOMEONE

You're in the quiet now.

The world feels wrong.
Too still.
Too heavy.
Too final.

You've spent months or years living in constant motion, constant alertness, constant worry, constant caregiving.
And now, in one moment, the crisis ended — and the silence is deafening.

Grief comes in waves that don't make sense.
One minute numb.
One minute shattered.
One minute relieved.
One minute guilty for being relieved.
One minute angry at everything.
One minute grateful for the peace.
One minute gasping for air.

This is normal.

All of it.

You didn't just lose a person.
You lost a role.
A purpose.
A routine.
A daily identity that shaped your entire world.

Your body doesn't know the caregiving is over.
Your brain still waits for calls, falls, and emergencies
that will never come.
Your heart still tries to protect someone who is no
longer here.

Let me tell you what no one else will say out loud:

You did enough.
You were enough.
You loved them enough.

Even on your worst days.
Even when you lost your patience.
Even when you felt trapped or resentful or broken.
Even when you prayed for relief and hated yourself
for wanting it.

You walked someone through a disease that takes

everything — and you stayed.
You stayed when it was hard.
You stayed when it hurt.
You stayed long after the version of them you knew
was gone.

YOUR LOVE OUTLASTED DEMENITA.

Their death is not your failure.
Their death is the end of the disease — not a
reflection of anything you did or didn't do.

You carried them farther than most people will ever
understand.

And now, it's your turn to rest.
Your turn to breathe.
Your turn to fall apart if you need to.
Your turn to remember who you were before this
began.

Healing will not be quick.
It will not be linear.
It will not look the way anyone expects.

But it will come.

And when it does, you will realize something true

and deep:

You did something extraordinary.
You loved someone through hell.
You walked them to peace with your own two
hands.
You were the last calm, the last touch, the last
familiar voice in a world that betrayed them.

That is sacred.
That is beautiful.
That is forever.

I'm proud of you.
I hope someday you're proud of yourself, too.

EPILOGUE
THE LAST WORDS YOU DESERVE — AFTER THE HARDEST JOURNEY YOU NEVER ASKED FOR

There's a moment at the end of every dementia journey that no one talks about.

The world gets quiet.
The emergencies stop.
The schedule that once ruled your life disappears.
And you're left standing there with a heart full of love,
a body full of exhaustion,
and a silence that feels too big for one person to hold.

You look back and realize you survived things you never imagined you could.
You stepped into realities you didn't choose.
You made decisions no one prepared you for.
You carried someone through the darkest, most vulnerable chapter of their life.

And even when you doubted yourself…
even when you felt like you were failing…
even when you were exhausted, frustrated, grieving,
resentful, devoted, terrified, hopeful —
you kept showing up.

That is love in its strongest form.

Dementia didn't get the final say.
Love did.

If you are reading these words after the journey…
or in the middle of it…
or before you even know what's coming…

I want you to know this:

Nothing about what you did — or are doing — is
small.
Nothing about the way you care is ordinary.
Nothing about the way you love is forgettable.

The world will never fully understand what
caregivers carry.
But I do.
And I wrote this book for you.

To give you language.

To give you truth.
To give you tools.
To give you something real in the middle of
something devastating.

And to remind you, now and always:

I f'n hate dementia — but your love did what the
disease never could:
it stayed.

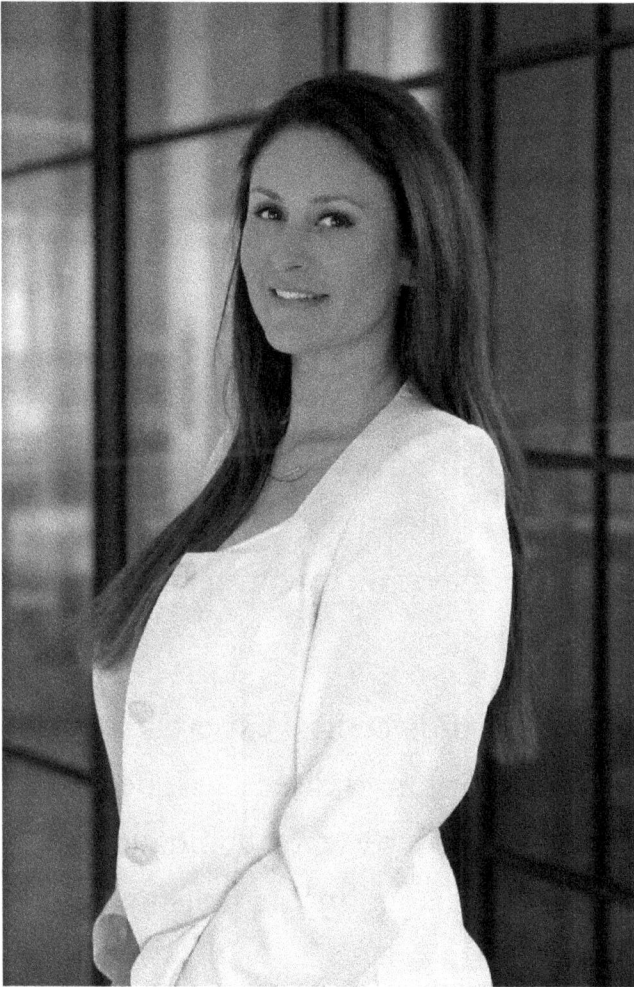

ABOUT THE AUTHOR

Ashley Ivy is a speech-language pathologist with advanced training in dementia care and caregiver support. She holds a Master's degree in Communication Disorders from Louisiana State University Health Sciences Center and maintains national certification through the American Speech-Language-Hearing Association (ASHA) with her Certificate of Clinical Competence (CCC-SLP).

Ashley has spent most of her professional career working in long-term care, alongside individuals living with dementia and the families who loved them. Through this work, she has witnessed firsthand how dementia reshapes lives, relationships, and identities — and how caregivers are often left to navigate it with far too little honesty or support.

Her approach blends clinical expertise with compassion, humor, and directness, because she believes caregivers deserve real guidance — not watered-down explanations or polished platitudes.

Outside of her professional life, Ashley is an extremely proud mother to her son, Preston, and a devoted animal lover. Her dogs have often worked alongside her over the years, becoming quiet sources of comfort, connection, and unexpected joy in dementia care settings.

Born and raised in Louisiana, Ashley now resides in

Texas and remains deeply committed to advocating for people who cannot always advocate for themselves — something she has done instinctively for as long as she can remember.

I F'n Hate Dementia is her way of standing beside caregivers in the hardest moments of the journey — with clarity, empathy, and the reminder that they are not alone.

www.ingramcontent.com/pod-product-compliance
Lightning Source LLC
Chambersburg PA
CBHW062050270326
41931CB00013B/3011